BARE

First published in 2015 by
Liberties Press
140 Terenure Road North | Terenure | Dublin 6W
T: +353 (1) 405 5701| www.libertiespress.com | E: info@libertiespress.com

Trade enquiries to Gill & Macmillan Distribution
Hume Avenue | Park West | Dublin 12
T: +353 (1) 500 9534 | F: +353 (1) 500 9595 | E: sales@gillmacmillan.ie

Distributed in the United Kingdom by
Turnaround Publisher Services
Unit 3 | Olympia Trading Estate | Coburg Road | London N22 6TZ
T: +44 (0) 20 8829 3000 | E: orders@turnaround-uk.com

Distributed in the United States by
Casemate-IPM
22841 Quicksilver Dr | Dulles, VA 20166
T: +1 (703) 661-1586 | F: +1 (703) 661-1547 | E: ipmmail@presswarehouse.com

ISBN: 978-1-910742-05-1
2 4 6 8 10 9 7 5 3 1

A CIP record for this title is available from the British Library.

Cover design by Karen Vaughan – Liberties Press
Internal design by Liberties Press

Printed and Bound in India by Thomson Press India Limited.

BARE

Irish Women's
Sexual Fantasies

Julianne Daly

For all the women who submitted their stories,
but especially the ones who did not

Contents

Foreword

Shawna Scott
Sex Siopa

As the American owner of a progressive Ireland-based online sex shop, one question I get asked more than almost any other is, 'So how does Ireland compare to America in terms of sexuality and sexual liberation?' When I hear this, I sometimes wonder if the questioner is looking for a confirmation bias, someone from the outside to say, 'Yes. I'm afraid it's true. Irish people suffer from a terminal case of repression, and Americans are over there in a circle giving each other erotic massages while sipping tantric lattes.'

However I don't really know if I can answer that question with the complexity it deserves. When I told my boyfriend's father that I was contributing to a book about Irish women's sexuality, he kindly reminded me, 'You're totally unqualified to write this piece. You didn't grow up here, and you certainly didn't live through a time when the Church had complete control of the country.'

I kind of agree with him. There is no way I could speak on behalf of all Irish women and say definitively that they are one way or another. To do so would be foolish and ignorant. While oppression from the British and the Church has most certainly shaped the cultural landscape of the country, the women I encounter in my work do not fit into any typical box or demographic. The women that I speak to come who come to Sex Siopa come here for a wide variety of different reasons. In the past week alone, I've received emails and phone calls from women all over the country. One was a university student, a first-time buyer, who had no idea where to begin or what kind of toy would suit her. Another was a woman who suffers from vaginismus and was referred to me by her physiotherapist. One woman wanted to know what the best vibrator was for someone post menopause. I had another customer who gave her submissive boyfriend a shopping list, because she was far too much of a goddess to be dealing with online shopping. She's kind of my hero now.

With such a broad spectrum in just a seven-day period, I would argue that there is greater diversity in female sexuality here in Ireland than there are differences between Irish and American female sexuality, but, sadly, we've gotten a raw deal from our national media, who have a terrible habit of depicting women either as 'lovely girls' or scantily-clad photocall models hanging out in St Stephen's Green, and nothing in between.

Despite this, in many ways, the Irish are a lot more liberal and progressive than we give ourselves credit for. Take, for example, our average age of first marriage, compared to America. According to a report from the Central Statistics Office in 2013, the average age for women in Ireland to get married is 32.6. However when you look at the US census, you get a radically different picture. In my home state of Washington, it's twenty-six. In the Mormon-dominant state of Utah, it's twenty-three!

I grew up in a conservative pocket of an otherwise decidedly liberal state. And, while urban Seattle lies just forty minutes north of my parents' home in the town of Puyallup, it seemed almost impossible to escape the small-town culture. The girls I grew up with – and even I – sometimes had very narrow plans for our lives. We'd go to college, meet the man of our dreams there, and get married after graduation. When I was in my final year in school, I argued with my twenty-one-year-old boyfriend, because he was still living with his parents and not going to college. This was unheard of in our town at the time. *How could he possibly be marriage material if he doesn't have his own place?* I thought to myself . . . at eighteen.

It's pretty clear from looking at the census data that one of the reasons why the age of first marriage in some areas is so low is pressure from religious institutions to stay chaste until marriage. I have friends from school who have openly told me that the reason they got married so young was because they couldn't wait any longer to have sex. Purity rings and virginity pledges were commonplace in my school. If you ever wondered where the right-wing Catholic think tanks here in Ireland get their playbook from, look no further than the megachurches and the millennial youth groups of America.

Another surprising fact is that Irish people may have more sexual partners in their lifetimes than Americans do. In 2011, the Centers for Disease Control released a survey that showed that American men slept with an average of seven partners in their lifetimes and women only four (though it must be said I am not entirely swayed by their data, as they only counted opposite-sex partners for the survey). In contrast, in 2013, the *Herald* and TodayFM conducted a survey that found that Irish people in their thirties have had an average of eight sexual partners. Another survey, quoted by the *Irish Independent* in 2010, put the number at eleven.

But the more the Internet connects the world, the more I see our two cultures melt together: Tinder and OKCupid are the preferred dating apps of choice in both countries; thanks to Netflix, much of our film and television is the same; people watching porn are generally all going to the same websites. Over the past ten years, we have begun to perceive the world through the same filters as our American counterparts. While the idea of the tech industry homogenising the international community scares the bejaysus out of me, I can also see the good it has done. Blogs, forums, Twitter, and social media are being used for sexual education and to start sexual movements across the globe. When reproductive rights stories come out in the States, we hear about it here.

Julianne Daly

Equally, our marriage referendum has been talked about all over the world.

Cultures merging and becoming homogenous between countries is sometimes seen as a bad thing, and I can understand why – nobody wants everywhere to be the same, with the same shops, brands and looks everywhere. But as the differences between countries decline and barriers to communication are removed, something wonderful also happens. Our 'community', and the people with which we identify, becomes defined by who we are and who we know, and not necessarily by where we are. If you are a straight person in a heteronormative culture, that's not a big deal. But if you are not – if you are LGBTQ, asexual, kinky, non-monogamous or anything else – the feeling of connection that a global culture can give you, and the sense of belonging to a community of like-minded individuals is invaluable. Smaller niche groups can share experiences and knowledge globally and learn from one another and, as this process continues, I think we'll see that there is a much greater difference between individual women's sexual interests in any given country than there are differences between, for example, Irish and American female sexuality.

Female sexuality is much broader than many people realise, and we have the science to back this up. There is a great book called *What Women Want*, by Dr Jesse Bering. The wide variety of female desires covered in the scientific research he highlights is truly amazing, and you should all go read it after you finish this book. The parallels between the fantasies described by Irish women in *Bare* and some of what science is telling us about female desire and its range is quite fascinating. A lot of those studies were done in the US, so again – this shows us that we're similar in the vastness of our range of sexual interests.

I am so delighted to see a book like *Bare* being published in Ireland. It is rare to see a depiction of Irish women as three-dimensional, fully formed sexual beings, with unique thoughts, fantasies and desires, and even rarer to hear those stories told from the perspectives of the women themselves. My hope is that this book will not only serve as erotic entertainment, but encourage more women across all age groups to explore their sexuality and start conversations with their partners about what they're into.

★

Sex Siopa is Ireland's first health-and-design-focused sex shop. It is owned and operated by Shawna Scott, who started it as a pop-up shop around Dublin at markets and events, and by supplying toys to friends directly. Shawna is in equal parts excited and saddened that Sex Siopa is the first Irish retailer dedicated to providing only toys and accessories that are bodysafe, and hopes that it will help to bring change to the industry and a push for better-designed products as part of a grassroots movement happening worldwide.

Introduction

I am known among my friends and acquaintances as someone who will talk about anything. I like to discuss the
undiscussed and name the elephant in the room. However,
even I find it difficult to talk about my sexual fantasies. It
just feels like a step too far, even when in the company of
my best friends, never mind in polite company. Even one of
my closest female friends, who is similarly open and honest,
stopped me in my tracks as I told her about this book. She
assured me that there was no way I would be getting a story
from her – some things are just private. When I spoke to
other people about bringing these stories together, their
reactions were varied. Most were full of enthusiasm and
said they would definitely submit their fantasies. Some were
a bit taken aback, and made it very clear that they wouldn't
be contributing. After two months of work, encouraging
people to submit stories, I only had twenty. While people

may be busy and time may be precious, I suspect this was, at least partly, a reflection of our discomfort in talking about sex and our sexual fantasies. One person started the survey and, when they got to the question asking for their fantasy, they wrote, 'Sorry, I just can't!' It wasn't until the media got wind of a book about Irish women and sex that word got out and the stories came flooding in.

When I mention the book to Irish men, they are fascinated. One of my friends expressed concern for the Irish male. He said that if they find out that Irish women are highly sexed after all, they will feel like failures, sexually, as that isn't their experience. Several men mention it to me every time we meet, asking me when it will be published. It seems to have piqued their interest. Clearly it's not just women who want to read it.

We hope that by bringing together the sexual fantasies of these Irish women, we can start a conversation about sex, and how women in this country think about it. Sex isn't simply what we see on television and in films or read about in books, but a universal experience made individual by each person's own proclivities. What each person finds arousing can be unique, and should be celebrated as such.

These stories were mostly collected anonymously through an online survey. Some were emailed. Several women contacted me afterwards to express their enthusiasm for the book. One of the contributors said:

'I am a highly sexual woman and often feel led to believe that I am in the minority – but surely that can't be the case! Not many of my friends talk openly about sex. Particularly after marriage, it seems, it can become a taboo subject. I can't wait for your book to hit the shelves!'

Another contributor said: 'I'm thrilled that someone is writing this book! Hope the process goes well, looking forward to reading it when it comes out!' Another added: 'I look forward to reading about the real thoughts women have. It's about time we embraced our inner naughtiness and dismissed preconceived ideas of women and sex.'

It seems there is a real hunger to know what other women are thinking about sex. Some women talked about not feeling normal. Others worried that there was something wrong with them, as heterosexuals, fantasizing about other women. Based on the submissions we received, Irish women fantasize about all sorts of things. Most of the women have never played out their fantasies in real life, though some of them toy with the idea of doing so. For most, the fantasies are imaginary, arousing scenarios normally kept to themselves – until now.

This book contains over a hundred sexual fantasies from over a hundred Irish women. Forty percent of our contributors were aged between eighteen and twenty-nine. The next biggest group were women in their thirties, who made up thirty-five percent of the contributors. Twenty-one percent of our contributors were in their forties, and three contributors were in their fifties. We had one story from a woman in her sixties.

Our contributor had a range of different sexual orientations. While eighty-one percent described themselves as heterosexual, thirteen percent identified as bisexual and almost five percent as lesbian.

Some of the stories have been edited to correct grammar and punctuation, or to make them clearer or more readable. Overall though, I have strived to maintain their original form. Most of the women have opted to use pseudonyms, but have given information pertaining their age, sexual preferences and so on.

When I began reading through the submissions my cheeks certainly flushed, and I felt quite giddy in anticipation of the end result. The stories were varied in tone, length and type of fantasy. I hope the book makes your cheeks flush, even just a little.

Infidelity

Polly-Ann

Polly-Ann is a heterosexual woman in her forties. She describes her sex drive as very high. She usually fantasizes before having sex and usually about men she knows, or her partner. She fantasizes about work colleagues, her friend's husbands and, in particular, her divorced next-door neighbour. She is married. Women also sometimes appear in her fantasies.

My husband has taken the kids away for the weekend. I had to work so I didn't go with them. As I am coming home from work, I meet my gorgeous forty-four-year-old divorced neighbour coming home too. We chat outside for half an hour and, as it starts to rain, he suggests we go into his place.

I can tell he is enjoying the company. I have already told him that I'm home alone this weekend. Eventually we open a bottle of wine, then another. I'm in a silk blouse and a knee-length work skirt. The conversation turns to sex – he says he hasn't had sex for three years since his wife left him. When I tell him I have only ever had sex with my husband, and regret not having enjoyed myself more before I was married, he suggests we have a one-off night of crazy passion. He is desperate to unload himself inside a woman, to feel her wetness and smell her odour. I could then fulfil my fantasy about having sex with another man. I let him persuade me a bit and then agree. We go upstairs. He takes off my blouse and black bra, and slowly licks my erect nipples. I'm boiling over. Even though I'm scared and guilty I can't stop myself. He takes off his shirt and then peels off his jeans. I take down his Y-fronts, allowing his bulging penis to rise quickly on its release. He takes off my knickers and starts to lick my inner thighs. This was a massive fantasy of mine that my husband did once – I just can't seem to ask him to do again. He goes on for ten minutes or so, and then his tongue enters my dripping wet vagina. The feeling is like nothing I've ever experienced. I push his head hard into me, then I pull him up until he's straddling me. He starts to push his penis though my breasts, its large head teasing my lips. I can just about lick its tip with my tongue. I can smell it. He goes faster and faster, and eventually covers my face in semen. Thankfully, I haven't cum yet, as this would disgust me if I was finished, so I lick in what I can reach. After forcing his fingers as far as he can into my vagina he is then amazingly ready to go again. He plunges his penis into me, deep and fast, again and again. I explode with an orgasm of galactic proportions. We lie there for a while, and after twenty minutes start all over again with me on top. I've never said this out loud, it's strange to write it out. I have to go to the bathroom now and lock the door or I will explode!

Dearbhla

Dearbhla is a heterosexual woman in her forties. She used to fantasize while having sex, but now it's just when she's alone – usually before she goes to sleep at night or before a lazy afternoon nap. She loves going to bed during the afternoon and getting naked on her own. She doesn't watch porn, but often fantasizes about characters from TV shows or movies.

There's one particular fantasy I have over and over again – it always does it for me. It features a young man who lives in the neighbourhood. He is about twenty years old and American (we're all American, it's like a TV show). I'm a sexy, married, more mature woman with a bit of a cougar thing going on. In my fantasy, I am at home and, for some reason, he cums to the house (he might be a gardener or something) and is surprised to find me there. He is very inexperienced but really well hung. He is broad-shouldered with sandy brown hair, and is not yet confident in his manliness. I'm there to teach him how to really make love to a woman. He walks in and sees me there and is taken aback. I can see how he is looking at me. I know he finds me really attractive and probably thinks about me when he masturbates. I know he's thought about having sex with me, and this is something that really turns me on – that he finds me so irresistible.

Of course, in my fantasy there are no flabby bits on my body, and my breasts are still as perky as a twenty-year-old's. I have a great cleavage (in my fantasy, not in real life) and I lean down as he talks to me so that he can get a good look. I am wearing silky red underwear under a silk robe and looking pretty hot. I walk up really close to him, run my index finger down his chest and ask him if he likes what he sees. He is at once flustered and aroused. He tries to act cool, but I can feel him getting hard as I stand there close to him. I lean in and kiss him, and he kisses back. He looks around nervously, but I assure him that my husband is away and won't be back till the next day. I lead him upstairs and tell him to relax. He tries to talk, but I rest my fingers against his lips. We share a deep, long kiss, and I feel him put his hands on me for the first time. My whole body is filled with electricity.

His jeans are bulging as I rip off his T-shirt, exposing his broad, muscular shoulders and tanned skin. He lifts me so I can wrap my legs around him, then slowly lowers me onto the bed. He tells me he has never done anything like this before, but I tell him to relax – that I'll show him what to do. I love looking at my breasts in their ruby-red lace, and at our bodies as the grind together. He lies on his back and I straddle him. I open his jeans slowly, driving him crazy. Once his jeans are off I start to kiss his upper leg, teasing him until I have his cock in my mouth. He is bucking and grinding so hard I stop so that he doesn't cum too soon. All the while he is begging me not to stop. I take his hand and place it on my red lace pants. His fingers soon find the right spot with my guidance, and I begin to move with the waves of pleasure going through my body.

I fling myself on my back and say, 'Fuck me . . . Now.' He is only thrilled to oblige, as he is hard as a rock and I've driven him crazy. He enters me and we both shout in ecstasy and I cum very soon after that – the most amazing, head-blinding, intense orgasm ever. Flippin' hell I wouldn't mind acting out that fantasy should the opportunity arise.

Chris

Chris is a heterosexual woman in her thirties. She rates herself as a good lover. She enjoys sex with her husband but never fantasizes about him. Her fantasies are almost always about men she knows or exotic female strangers. Her current favourite is a friend's brother who she sees from time to time. There is definitely sexual chemistry between them, but she would never be unfaithful to her husband in real life.

My friend has this brother who I have known for several years. We often meet when he is home from overseas. He is in a long-term relationship – as am I – but I always notice that I pay a little extra attention to my appearance when I know I'm going to see him. I regularly fantasize about what it would be like to spend a day with him in bed.

In my fantasy, he is home for an extended holiday and my husband is away on business. He is staying in a hotel in the city, and I am up for the day shopping. He texts me early that morning saying he heard I was in Dublin, and asking whether I fancy meeting for lunch. I agree, of course, and rush to the nearest make-up counter for a subtle but perfect look. After I get a quick blow-dry and some sexy new underwear, I casually stroll into the restaurant where he is already waiting for me. We kiss on the cheek and it is electric. We both know something is going to happen. My heart is beating so fast, blood is flowing to my vagina and I feel myself begin to warm up. I want to fuck this man so much. I just can't believe this is happening. Never once in my fantasy do I feel any guilt about my husband – it's pure fantasy-land, so I don't go there. We spend lunch talking about everything and nothing, with short pauses where we just stare at each other and smile, taking each other in.

As we leave the restaurant, we don't even mention what we are about to do. We silently make our way towards his hotel, not touching in case we meet anyone we know. I just want to rip his clothes off at this point. We arrive at the hotel and can't get upstairs quickly enough. The elevator doors close, and he immediately pushes me up against the wall, kissing me passionately. As the door opens, he grabs my waist as we wordlessly make our way to his room. He is so frantic he can barely open the door. Once the door closes, we break loose, all inhibitions going out the window.

We do it like you see it in the movies. We kiss against the door of the room and rip each other's clothes off. He pushes me down on the bed and, half-clothed, we take it a little slower, just to make it last. I am wearing raunchy, slutty underwear, completely at odds with the conservative dress and pearls that cover it. My nipples are hard, and he sucks them with so much intensity that it almost hurts. He stands up to take off his trousers, his penis hard and enormous. He stands over me with his hands on the bed either side of me. He looks me up and down, taking in every detail before he devours me. He kneels down and slowly takes my knickers off, kissing my pussy gently, driving me crazy. We haven't spoken a word since we left the restaurant and we still say nothing, not wanting to break the spell. His tongue flicks between my folds, making me even wetter. I can't wait any more. I pull him up from his knees and push him back onto the bed. I take him in my mouth and watch as he is overcome with pleasure. It makes me feel like a wonderful lover and the sexiest I have ever been. I straddle him and we watch each other as he slowly enters me. The intensity is mind-blowing, and we both cum together, screaming our heads off, not caring if anyone hears us.

Thea

Thea is a heterosexual woman in her late teens or twenties. She has a high sex drive and regularly reads erotica. She usually fantasizes when she is alone, and the subject of her fantasies varies. Quite often it'll be one of her adult students – she feels that the teacher-student power dynamic always adds a little something.

My fantasies vary a lot, both in terms of scenarios and the

people involved. A lot of the time there's a large group of people in a dark, glamorous room, like a sex party. At first I'm just watching other people as they get carried away, but then a hot guy comes out of nowhere – maybe he's been watching too, or maybe he's been watching *me*, I don't know. He grins at me with this wicked look in his eyes, then pulls me up against him in a scorching kiss. We tumble into a pile of other bodies and everyone from that point on is wild and totally uninhibited.

At the moment, I mostly fantasize about a friend I met in Italy. He lives abroad and already has a girlfriend, unfortunately, but the chemistry between us is incredible. He's not my usual type at all, but we can talk about absolutely anything – including sex – very openly. He's very charming, intelligent and physical, and more than a little bit cocky. Intoxicating. I've had an almost-certainly doomed crush on him since we met, seeing as he lives abroad and is already taken, but the chemistry between us is just too strong for my imagination to ignore.

We meet again after months apart, both single, and he can't take his eyes off me. We go for drinks, or dinner, or dancing, and talk about life, the universe and everything. But after a few hours, a few drinks and more than a few scorching glances, he gives in to it and kisses me, crushing me against him like nothing else matters. We take a taxi back to his place or mine, and the moment the door shuts behind us, he slams me up against it. Our bodies are pressed together, and we are necking like teenagers. We nearly rip each other's clothes we're so keen to get them off, and we barely make it to the bedroom before he throws me backwards onto the mattress, pinning my wrists above my head and going to town on me. It's hard and fast and unbelievably intense. We both know there'll be plenty of time for tenderness later; we're not going anywhere. It's the desperate release of all that tension and chemistry after so long, with both of us trying to remain on our best behaviour – that's what makes it really intoxicating.

Kym

Kym is a bisexual woman in her forties. She regularly reads erotica. She sometimes reminisces about past lovers, and often thinks about her fantasies when she's running. This may be partly due to the fact that she imagines running with an imaginary personal trainer, with whom she gets into all sorts of sexcapades, usually initiated by the rubbing of a sore muscle. Her post-run showers are very enjoyable. She is married, and usually fantasizes about particularly exciting past encounters.

I am lucky to have had some great sex over the years, so I tend to reminisce rather than fantasize, though sometimes the reminiscences are a little bit enhanced by fantasy! After completing my Leaving Cert, I went to college in Britain. I was still going out with my boyfriend from school, and not looking for anyone in university.

While working in the students' union, I met Joe, who was a bouncer and fellow student. He tried to chat me up over several weeks. I loved my boyfriend and wanted to stay faithful, but the relentless flirting was very flattering. He had a way of staring at my body that would get us both hot. He would unashamedly display his erection to me.

I couldn't believe that I could have that effect on someone without even touching them. I began to inflame him even more by dressing more provocatively. I would bend over, giving him an eyeful, or show off my ass in a short skirt, under the pretence of just going about my work. I pretended I didn't realise I was flashing him, and I would always knock back his advances. I even told him about my boyfriend back home. Harmless flirting wasn't cheating, after all.

Joe was a mature student in his early thirties and much more sexually experienced than I. Rather than using the normal cheesy chat-up lines, Joe worked to dispel my Catholic hang-ups around sex. 'Having sex is just like satisfying any other bodily need, like hunger or thirst', he would say. I was brought up to believe that you had to be profoundly in love before even considering having sex. Joe made me change my mind completely, he taught me to enjoy sex on its own, without the emotional baggage of love. I eventually succumbed to him. It turned out that Joe was excellent at cunnilingus and thoroughly enjoyed it. Up until then, I had been too full of Catholic guilt to let my Irish boyfriend try this with me.

Tilly

Tilly is a heterosexual woman in her late teens or twenties. She has a high sex drive and considers herself to be a good lover. She fantasizes both when she is alone and during sex.

I usually fantasize about someone famous, Charlie Hunnam is a good one. I don't mind a bit of 50 Cent either. I like to fantasize about a man that can and will take control. With Charlie, it's more his character Jax that I imagine, rather than the actor himself. It's sometimes more the body that I'm attracted to than the face. I imagine acting out scenes with Jax when I'm kissing him. I play out little scenarios in my head.

My fantasies often include hot sex and ripping clothes, not being able to take our hands off each other, and being thrown down onto the bed, stairs, couch or table. He is usually a strong, dominant male lifting me up, and we go from there. But before that there's lots of flirting. He has a girlfriend sometimes and breaks off with her to have me. He wants me, but I won't go there because I know he is taken. It makes the flirting more fun. You want what you can't have.

Marie-Claire

Marie-Claire is a heterosexual woman in her thirties. She has a low sex drive and mostly fantasizes when she is alone. She is married, and the subject of her fantasy is usually a man or woman that she knows.

For some reason, my fantasies almost always involve someone telling me they've always wanted me. It's like I need the adoration in order to feel aroused. I often fantasize about one of my friends' husbands. I often don't even fancy him but, for some reason, in my fantasies, I want him to want me. In my fantasy, we are away at some hotel, and just happen to be in the same city at the same time. No one will know. No one – including my husband – will ever find out, so no one will get hurt. It's our secret. We are always half-naked, and the foreplay is always fast and desperate, ripping off each other's clothes. I am always wearing red underwear, and my body is toned and tanned. He always gets turned on when he sees my breasts in this beautiful underwear. He is hard as a rock, wild with desire and can't wait to have me. We never get fully naked – he doesn't have the self-control to wait until all my clothes are off. I cum almost as soon as he enters me. If he or his wife ever knew I'd had these thoughts, I would be mortified!

BDSM
Bondage, Discipline and Sadomasochism

Ailish

Ailish is a heterosexual woman in her forties. She usually fantasizes at night before she goes to sleep. She has a high sex drive when she's in a relationship. However, when she is alone, her fantasy life depends on her menstrual cycle. She usually fantasizes about her current lover or an imaginary man. Sometimes this man is an ex, but never a film star or celebrity.

Your hand on my hair is sensual but also a gesture of control. My breath freezes in anticipation as you speak, my nerves tingling from the timbre of your voice, my body responding to your direct gaze, your confident stance. I press against you and you don't respond, my wanton nature amusing you. I suppress a sigh of frustration, and you tighten your grip on my hair. My scalp is pinched, and the sharp pain makes me gasp. You hold my gaze, observing and enjoying the fracturing of my control, my mask slipping. I'm playing at being a grown-up, and my dry mouth gives away my nerves. I can see the other people in the room fucking and it's turning me on watching them and being here. You let me watch for a few minutes as you keep a tight grip on my hair with one hand, the other hand pinching and stroking my nipples, which melts me.

I'm feeling gratitude. I'm horny, and I'm enjoying the delicious sinking feeling of submitting to your will. You step closer. The hardness of your cock makes me gasp. I rub myself along its length, maintaining eye contact. I really want you to fuck me, just like all those other sluts. I'm nothing special after all. You feel my soft, swollen cunt, brushing the wet hair and parting my lips. You ask me what I want and I can't say it. You kick my legs apart, which makes me gasp again. As your strong fingers finish spreading my wet cunt, you order me to get down on my knees. I comply, mouth getting wet, lips swelling, eyes wide, sluttishly eager to please you.

You hold my face as I lick my stickiness from your fingers. My eagerness freezes as you indicate that I should open my mouth. I open my mouth wide and stick out my tongue, and you slap your thick cock onto it.

'There's a good girl,' you say. 'Now suck my cock.'

I'm compliant before my brain even catches up, licking the tip and sucking you deep into my mouth, the head pressing into my throat with every stroke. I'm trying my best moves, and trying to keep my distance so you don't choke me.

You grab hold of my head tight and start fucking my face. My muffled grunts and attempt to back away are futile. Your grip is strong and your cock slams into the back of my throat hard enough to make me gag and salivate. The thick head of your cock spreads my mouth open and covers the back of my throat, pushing deep. I can feel the force of your hips behind each thrust, the wet tightness makes you harder and you push forcefully through my lips, stretching and battering my mouth. You pull out and watch as I gasp for breath. Looking up shakily, I thank you.

'Good girl,' you say.

You grip my hair again and I open my mouth, eyes down.

'Feel your tits,' you order, and I obey, squeezing my breasts and pulling hard at the nipples, stretching them out so you can see what a good slut I am.

'Good,' you say. 'Now open up, like a good girl.'

You resume fucking my mouth, thrusting deep. I have no other thought than keeping my wet mouth steady. For me, all thoughts are gone except my breathing, the heat in my cunt and a desire to please you.

My succubus nature takes over and the hunger for cock rises, the hunger to taste sticky, salty cum. I start moaning in pleasure even as I gag and leak spit as you use my mouth. My body is in charge now, I'm even more horny and, momentarily, I wish I was riding you, slamming down hard onto your cock. I pinch my tits harder, excited, feeling my back arch, my ass sticking out.

You withdraw again, gripping your hard length, sticky spit dripping from my mouth onto the head of your cock, and I know you're close. You see the mix of endurance, subservience and sheer pleasure in my face as I anticipate your orgasm, my tongue ready to receive your cum.

You grip the sides of my head roughly and fuck my mouth mercilessly. I'm gagging and retching, glad of my empty stomach as I gasp for breath and choke as your cock slides in and out, in and out, deep into my wet, tight throat. You're losing yourself in the moment, and you cum, your cock bulging in my throat, flooding, choking, your eyes open as you watch me choke on your cock, as it pushes silvery cream down my throat, my gagging, swallowing sounds pleasing you. I moan with pleasure as I savour each droplet of your cum, my tongue licking the head, sucking the still-hard shaft, making you moan even more as I milk you, sucking every last drop.

Jillian

Jillian is a heterosexual woman in her late teens or twenties. She fantasizes before sex, during sex and when alone. She is currently single, and doesn't fantasize about anyone in particular, but she does have a particular scenario that she replays.

There's a girl in a bar having a few drinks with friends. She catches the eye of a guy standing nearby, and he plays it cool and looks away. They get chatting later in the night and end up going home together. They are strangers, but the chemistry between them is electric. She knows he wants to fuck her brains out and she absolutely loves it. She loves having people want her, fantasizing about what they will do to her. When they get home, he is very rough. He pushes her angrily up against the wall, immediately ripping her underwear off from under her dress. He wants to dominate her, and she is in her element. He pulls her hair hard as he bites and kisses her neck, licking her all the way down to her breasts. She wants to put up a fight. She likes to feel like what's happening shouldn't really be happening. She likes to feel like it's wrong, so resisting his hard cock inside her adds to her pleasure. Through her resistance, he gets even rougher, and finally forces her hands above her head, holding her strongly while trying to force his cock inside her. She is wet and turned on as he teases her with the top of his dick. After more resistance and fighting, he pushes his cock inside her hard.

Sarah

Sarah is a heterosexual woman in her forties. She has submitted several fantasies for this book. She mostly fantasizes when she is alone, and it's usually about someone she knows. This man is a married friend of hers who she describes as tall, dark and gorgeous. She has known him since primary school and, back in their single days, they had a few sexual encounters. They remain good friends, and though she never wants to be in a relationship with him, he is getting even better looking with age. The first fantasy below is about him.

Usually in my fantasy, he has somehow acquired my spare house key. He comes in to my house in the middle of the night, and I wake up with him tenderly tying my hands to the bed. He whispers to me, 'I have always wanted you so badly'. He finishes tying up my hands, gently caressing my whole body, drinking in the effect his hands are having on me. His hands travel down to my clitoris, and he knows exactly what to do to make me cum. Just as I begin to cum, he enters me with his big throbbing cock, and fucks me like it's his last fuck in the world. I cum again. Then, before leaving the house he whispers, 'I'm holding onto your spare key. See you soon, sexy'.

A slightly more hard-core fantasy involves me being tied to a wheel in an S & M club, and being lightly whipped by passing strangers, both men and women. Then some devastatingly attractive female will step up to the wheel, swing it around so that I'm upside down, and proceed to lick me out and make me cum. This fantasy may be somewhat related to the horniness I get from inversions while practising yoga!

Beth

Beth, who is in her forties, describes herself as an 'edge dweller', a warrior of the heart and a passionate lover of free-

dom. She is the founder and director of Bliss Ireland and The Irish Festival of Erotic Art, as well as a co-founder and lead facilitator at 'Turas Fián'. Beth thinks of herself as a sexual being and doesn't like using labels to describe who she is attracted to, as she finds that it limits how others perceive her and how she can perceive herself. She doesn't really have relationships like most other people do. She doesn't enjoy monogamy, and prefers to give herself and those she is involved with total freedom to be and do as they please. That's not a licence for disrespect or a lack of commitment, but a gift of total and absolute freedom to be who and how they want to be, and to be fully and freely loved for that. She has been living in rural Ireland for the last fifteen years, having spent the previous fifteen living in the wild hearts of Dublin, Toronto and Belfast. She doesn't fantasize about having sex with people she is not actually involved with.

In the privacy of her temple, where they were to meet, he stood and waited, surrounded by the deep reds and rich burnt oranges of the plush and soft fabrics of the spacious room, intoxicated by the scents of sandalwood and jasmine. She had asked that he wear only a T-shirt and sweatpants, that he light the candles, turn off the lights and start the playlist loaded on her laptop and then stand, facing away from the door, in the middle of the room and not to move when she entered. He did as she asked, quite the uncomfortable role-reversal for him, but he trusted that she knew both of them individually, and the space between them that was their relationship, well enough to know what would work for them both.

He closed his eyes and allowed the hypnotic, somewhat-seductive music, new to his ears, wash over him in undulating waves, felt his shoulders slowly lower, the knot in his back unravel and his hips begin to feel loose and free. He stretched his arms over his head, hearing his back crack slightly as it arched, then heard the thump of her bare feet on the tiled floor walking towards the room in which he was waiting.

The door opened quietly and closed a moment later. He wondered if she'd cum in or not, but then heard the sound of something solid and hard being put on the wooden floor behind him. He felt her approach from behind, her hands lightly on his hips at first, then taking either side of his T-shirt with her fingertips, and slowly and gently moving it up his body. He understood it to mean that she wanted to take it off so he helped. She returned her hands to his hips and began to slide his sweatpants very slowly down over his hips, over his swelling cock and down his legs. He felt something cold against his skin and, flinching slightly, he jerked away but her hand grabbed his wrist and a quiet 'Shhhh' came from her lips. He stilled, returned to standing and clenched his jaw. The leather and steel restraints closed snugly around his wrists, holding his arms firmly behind his back. This was the first time he had ever allowed another to restrain him and, in that moment, he realised that he trusted her.

She stepped away from him and he heard her catch her breath slightly. He felt her warm breath – her mouth must have been an inch or so from his skin. She followed the touch of her breath with her nipples. He began to lean back into her, but she quickly moved away and he had to steady himself, erection rising, and she came close again, agonisingly slowly pressing her soft, ample breasts into his back, her nipples hard now.

When she placed her fingers and then palms of her hot hands on his shoulders, he shivered, erection jutting out now, as she moved slowly and deliberately down his body, caressing his back, shoulders and arms with her lips, breath, hair, breasts and fingertips. He moaned in pleasure. She remained quiet but he noticed her breath becoming laboured. She moved down his body, her warm and wet tongue gliding between the cheeks of his ass slowly as she moved down his legs and then stepped away from him. His balls ached for her now.

Hearing a soft swirl of fabric, he realised that she meant to blindfold him, so he let her; he had surrendered to her now. She left him untouched. Then, cock and balls throbbing, arms trapped behind his back, blindfolded, for what felt like minutes.

She came back, letting out a purr that came from the pit of her, and emanated through vibrating lips against his skin.

She circled him slowly, trailing cool fingertips and hot breath in a slow spiral down his body. She trailed fingers over his aching balls, deliberately avoiding his cock. As she finished circling him, she laid her hands on the fronts of his feet and pressed firmly. Then she lifted her left hand and replaced it with warm lips and feather-soft kisses, and did the same to his other foot.

His cock felt her first – the junction of her thighs, those soft, welcoming legs. Her lips feathered his chest with the lightest of kisses, hair brushing his nipples, breasts now caressing his skin. She allowed the tip of her tongue to lightly brush against his dripping cock tip for one agonising, blissful moment.

He was confused by desire, his head reeling from want, every skin cell alive and bursting with hunger for her. Then she was in front of him, on her knees. She pulled a little closer and he felt her belly and breasts against his knees and thighs. Her mouth must have been inches from his cock. He felt the hot breath, and his hips thrust forward. He wanted to be in her mouth, filling her as she liked him to, but as she moved back quickly. Fists, buttocks and jaw clenching and then relaxing, allowing the pleasure roll through him in waves, a wet tongue finally circled the tip of his cock. She leaned back and left him without her touch for a moment, and then wet, warm lips encircled the tip again. He heard her moan, the vibrations of her lips travelling down the shaft.

She was hungry for his cock, he could feel it. She took him deep into her throat, then reached around to his back and released his hands from their bondage. The restraints fell to the floor with a loud crash. She guided his hands to the back of her head while her lips tightened around his girth, her breasts pressed tightly to his thighs and her hands gripped his hips. Moans came from deep in her belly. 'Please cum in my mouth', she breathed quietly. Her words were his undoing and he gushed into her mouth, filling her throat. He heard her hungrily moan as the orgasm filled his entire body.

They were both quiet then, relaxed and stilled. Her

hands remained on his hips, and her lips stayed around his cock. She drank him into her, then licked her lips and washed him clean again. Eventually she slipped him out of her mouth completely, but he waited patiently, for this was still her scene. After a few minutes of silence she spoke in a deep voice with a deliberate tone.

'My love, I invoke the divine in you to me, for me, for you, for us and for all that is,' she said. 'I don't have need of you, I am full and complete without you, but I invite you to share with me because I want you to cum and enter this vortex of life with me, for us to adventure together. Please take off your blindfold now.' And he did, humbled by the obvious love, sincerity and devotion in her words. He opened his eyes and there she kneeled, naked, upright, back arched, neck long, arms raised, head bowed, hands open and cupped, holding a soft and elegant black leather collar with a solid platinum 'O' ring and buckle, the very one he'd chosen for her months ago.

Her gaze meeting his, resolute, proud, strong, determined and full of love. She said slowly and deeply, 'Peter, I invite you to anoint these lips, consecrate this flesh, join with me and consummate this sacred desire.'

With this she offered him the collar, and therefore herself . . .

Kathryn

Kathryn is a bisexual woman in her forties. She lives in rural Ireland and is currently in a relationship. She has a high sex drive.

She holds onto the bedpost with both hands, her hair covering her face. I slip my finger under the ribbons of her corset, feeling the way it binds her. Leaning into her, I run my lips over her shoulder, then take the ribbons in both hands and pull. She gasps, but doesn't speak. Her body is mine to play with, mine to share, if I want. I tighten the ribbons to where I want them. Her breath comes quickly. I run my fingers over the raw silk and downwards to the soft flesh below. She's perfect: her bum swells out, round and ripe, from beneath the lace, and her legs were made for the long silk stockings I gave her to wear. I pull a suspender and let it snap back onto her, as I watch her chest heave up and down with the promise of what is to come. I run my hands through her hair, gathering the tresses together – then fisting them behind her neck. I gently ease her around to look at me. I want her to know that she is mine. I want her to know that I know this, too. She drops her eyes, and her tongue darts to her lips.

There is a knock at the door, and a man comes in. She tries to turn away, tries to hide herself from him, but I shake my head. Releasing her hair, I spin my finger in the air, and she turns. Her fingers grip the very edge of the corset. She is nervous, but she wants to be there. I smooth my hands over her breasts and gently ease them up until her nipples show over the corset. Bullet-hard, they spring up, and I pinch one, just because I can. She lets out a small moan and I dip my head to kiss her. Her lips are soft, her mouth opens for me, and, as I kiss her, I run my hand over her hip, around the smooth underside of her belly and down, into the folds of her cunt. She's wet. Her muscles squeeze my fingers, needing more, but I stand back. Her eyes are wide, but, as I gesture, she kneels.

The man opens his zip and steps forward. I slide my fingers around the back of her neck, wiping her juices against her skin, then push my fingers into her hair again.

'Open,' I say, and she parts her lips for his cock. He slides into her mouth, pushing back into her throat, but I hold her hair, keeping her in place.

'Open,' I say again, a little firmer. She moves her knees, opening her legs for me.

'Again,' I say.

She closes her eyes as she sucks him, but I jerk her head, and she looks up at me. She has to know I am in control.

'Open,' I say, firmly. Watching me, she puts both hands on her buttocks, and opens. I nod. The man grunts, moving quicker. I ease her head towards him with each thrust, and she laps and sucks, and pulls on him with her mouth.

'You can cum on her face,' I say, 'or in her mouth.'

She blinks, but he's too far gone to stop, and he spills into her, thrusting deep as he comes.

'Swallow,' I tell her.

She gags slightly, but does as I say. When he pulls away, I let him go without a glance. She did well.

I smooth her hair back from her face, letting it fall onto her shoulders, but I do not move her hands. I go to the bed, and reach into my bag. She knows what is coming; she knows by the sound of the zip on the bag, by the pop of the lid of the lube. I run my fingers over the silicone, breathing in the sweet scent.

41

She's ready, and she holds my gaze as I nudge the plug into her ass. It's tight, but the lube oils her, and I feel her leaning back against me as I push it up inside her. 'Hold your hair', I say. She puts her hands up to her head and bunches her hair at the back of her neck. Her breasts pop up fully over the corset, and I flick her nipples with my fingers, catching the very tips. Then I pull her up to her feet, and let her stand with her back to the bedpost.

She licks her lips, ready to kiss me, but I ease her legs apart again. Her cunt is dripping wet and, as I push my fingers inside, I can feel the plug in her ass through the thin wall. She hears the buzz of the vibrator before I touch her with it, and she widens her legs, welcoming me.

'You see that door,' I say, as I press the vibe to her clit. I turn up the speed, and she clenches around my fingers. Gasping, she nods.

'If I wanted, I'd open that door right now.' Her breath comes quickly, and I push my hand further inside as she grips hold.

'I'd bring them in, one by one, and make you stand here and cum while they watched,' I say. 'They would see you with the plug up your ass, with your tits out, with your cunt dripping wet, and they would watch you cum for me, while they wait for you to suck them off.'

I lean my weight forward, knowing that as she presses herself back against the bedpost the plug is forced deeper inside her, knowing that she knows what I am doing. As her eyes roll back, as her hands fly up to grip the bedpost, I reach around and grip the plug, waiting until the last minute to pull it out, waiting for the muscles to snap back into place. Then, as she cries out, as her body shakes, I slam it back inside her, and she falls, panting, to her knees.

'Open,' I say, as the next man knocks at the door.

Abbi Rode

Abbi is a heterosexual woman in her thirties. She describes herself as having a very high sex drive. She regularly reads erotica and usually fantasizes about the last person she slept with, or someone she has had good sex with before. Both men and women feature in her fantasies, and two of her fantasies feature in this book.

He had mentioned that he was going to spank me properly. I'd been spanked before, but not properly, not like he was intending. I was also aware that he might be good at it, and I'd waited a long time to find out. It's exactly what I'd fantasized about. He's naked, I'm naked, we're on his bed. He's kneeling and his hands are free. He tells me to get on all fours. I do. He angles me around so that he has my head by his cock and his hand near my arse. He holds my head close to his cock. It's solid and fully erect, and I badly want it in my mouth. He knows this, and is toying with me. He calmly tells me what he's going to do to me and that I'm going to do what he says and with no mistakes, or he'll have to start again. He's going to spank me as I suck him off, and I'm not to break rhythm. I'm to count as he slaps me. I'm to thank him, and call him 'Sir'. I hate this and I love it. My heart is racing, and I know I'm wet.

He finally lets me have his cock in my mouth. He tells me that sometimes he'll let me do what I want to it, and sometimes he'll control it. He tells me that he'll make me gag on it, or force my head down and make me choke. This excites me more. I don't really know what's coming with either the spanking or the blow job; I have no control. All the pleasure is out of my hands, and all I can do is obey, and hope.

He lets me suck him for a little while as he explains how he wants it and what he expects of me. All the while he gently has one hand on the back of my neck, fingers curled in my hair but not forcing me to do anything. His other hand is a flat palm circling my arse: gently, softly, encouragingly. All my senses are heightened, waiting for him to strike. Will it be the mouth or the arse first? It feels like this goes on for an age, when in all likelihood it's not even two full minutes. He is stroking me with all the measured calm of an owner. But every delicate curl of his fingers in my hair, every warm, sweet rub of my arse piques my adrenaline with its ambiguous tenderness. What is coming? I am aching for him. I wish there was another one of him underneath me, licking me, eating me.

He takes his time, and the first move is to shove my head down hard onto his cock so that I gag. He holds me there just long enough, calling me a good girl in a darkly lustful, controlling tone. Just as he releases my head he wallops my arse for the first time. I barely have his cock out of my mouth in time to say the words. I struggle, both to catch my breath and to say the words. I hate them; this isn't who I am. But I want it. I want to be owned by him. I want to obey and at the same time rail against it. This is delicious torture. I want to surrender to his control. I want to trust that he will push me only so far. That he knows what he's doing. I don't have to think what to do, I don't have to guess, I don't have to do anything – I just have to obey and surrender to my own rising pleasure. I'm out of breath and have let the spit drip all down his solid cock as I manage to say: 'One. Thank you, Sir.'

The 'Sir' is the hardest part. I think he knows this. I cringe at this but in his polite and lovely way he convinced me that it was going to happen, and that I would do it. Conversations passed and moved on and once he had the agreement on the 'thank you', he introduced the notion that I would be calling him 'Sir'. Again I baulked at this, but he knew he had me, he knew I was going to do it, he knew I wanted it.

So I say it, and before I can catch my breath properly and he shoves my head back down onto his cock, makes a satisfied noise, and says 'Good'. He circles my arse with his hand and soothes where he's hit. He takes his time with the next smack, and comes down hard on my other arse cheek. Just before I go to release his cock to say the words, he shoves my head right onto it so that I deep throat him, holding me there for a second before releasing my head. Again I am choking as I say the words, but this time he calls me a good girl, and only runs his fingers through my hair as I go back to sucking it. I am wildly turned on.

Slaps three and four come in quick succession. If I wasn't half-choking I'd be heaving and barely able to breathe anyway. I am sucking him hungrily and he isn't controlling it –

it's just my mouth and tongue. He calls me a good girl, and tells me he knew I would be this obedient. He tells me that I'm a good little sub. He squeezes my arse cheeks and tells me they've come up nice and red. I am still sucking on his cock and just aching with every fibre in me to be fucked, to be touched, to be devoured. He knows this too. He asks me do I think I'm wet. *Oh God, please, please let him check*, I think. Please let him slide two fingers into me to find out. He does slide two fingers into me, and I am so wet for him. I clench onto them, gagging for them to stay there while I still have his rock-hard cock in my mouth, working it up and down.

But he isn't here to relieve me. No sooner has he got fingers in me for a few thrusts than he pulls them out and slaps me hard again. I stupidly wasn't expecting it. It was perfect. Again he pushes my head down onto his cock, making sure he's in control, fucking my face any way that he wants, using me as a toy. We eventually get to ten, and that's the end. I am past aroused – I am insane with need for him. I am blind with desire for his cock inside of me, and I finally get it. He pushes me face first onto the bed and ploughs into me.

Carole-Ann

Carole-Ann is a bisexual woman in her late teens or twenties. She has a low sex drive. She is currently single and mostly fantasizes when she is alone, about a friend of hers who is a 'bit of an idiot', whose looks make up for failings in personality.

I always see my fantasies from a third-person perspective, like a movie (a classy version, there are definitely filters at play). My arms are tied above me with something gentle and my partner is behind me. He is in total control as he rubs his hands all over my back and body. He touches me gently, not roughly in the way that so many Irish men seem to think is sexy. He moves to stand in front of me, then goes down on me as I wrap my legs around him. Soon he is holding me up, and I pull myself up using the ribbons tied round my wrists. While still holding me, he stands up and with him supporting me, we have sex, my legs wrapped tightly around him.

Harley

Harley is a heterosexual woman in her late teens or twenties. She regularly reads erotica, and normally has sexual fantasies when she is alone. At the moment she is enjoying fantasies about someone she fancies at work.

I am the boss in my office, but when it comes to the bedroom, I prefer for him to take full control. I walk in and he is standing there in the kitchen, waiting for me with hand restraints. Then he ties me to the kitchen table, before taking off his belt and whipping me across the back. I plead for him to stop. He says he is disgusted by me because I said I'd be home earlier than this. I don't apologise. He wraps his belt around my neck and ties it tight, practically holding me up by it, until my face starts turning blue. He lets me go just before I slip into unconsciousness, unzips his jeans and forces his cock down my throat. My eyes water as he pinches my nipples until they feel raw. He pours hot wax onto them, relishing my pained cries. I say something that he considers out of line, for which I get a smack across the face and my hair pulled back hard, making me look at him, as he makes me suck him off then cums all over my face. He ends by untying me and kissing me lovingly, so that I know he's my master, and that I love him more than I love myself.

Amy

Amy is a bisexual woman in her thirties. She is in a relationship and has a high sex drive. She has a lot of fantasies, generally surrounding BDSM, submission and objectification.

I have had one particularly potent and curious fantasy all my life. Since I can remember, I have been fascinated by transformation – transformation of size, shape and gender. Most often, however, I have had a fascination with cartoon-style transformation. The cartoonish idea of being flattened by a steamroller, a runaway rock or a cement block has always made me feel instantly aroused. The fantasy does not involve death or pain, but rather a miracle transformation from 3D to 2D – from human to object – in the space of a few seconds.

Being quite a bookish child, I would frequently read dictionary definitions of certain key words ('flatten', 'squash' and 'steamroll', for example) to get my fantasy started. It usually followed the same pattern, and it still does today. I am flattened by a lover, partner or friend 'for my own good'. Sometimes it is done to me suddenly without my knowledge, and sometimes I am aware in advance of it happening, but the former is the more frequent fantasy. Within moments, I realise that I love both the sensation and the inability to move. While flattened, I cannot speak or move, but I can see, hear and feel. Pleasure becomes intensified so as to be almost unbearable, and pain disappears, transmuted into a darker type of pleasure.

I am totally helpless, my lover can use me as anything he desires. This frequently includes a variety of household items – a sheet, a towel, a doormat. I am used in these states constantly, washed and ironed like a piece of laundry. Family and friends witness my humiliation and enjoy it, generally commenting that it 'suits me'. Ultimately, I end up remaining in my flattened form, generally through being re-inflated and given the option of being permanently flattened, or staying in my original form. I choose to be flattened and am once again pressed out, this time with no chance of escape.

My lover becomes my owner and I their object. By this point in the fantasy, I generally climax. Once the orgasm has passed, I tend to create a mental loophole where my lover actually misses me and chooses to return me to my 3D state. This fantasy has been with me since I can remember. I began to masturbate to it at the age of seven, but I had no idea what it was that I was doing until much later – I just enjoyed the sensations flooding into my body. My mind also alters during it and everything becomes about it – I can completely forget about any problems, troubles or worries until after I have climaxed.

For some years I ceased exploring it, as I began to believe that it was sick and unhealthy. But as I got older and more sexually experienced, I realised that the fantasy was harmless and important to me, and I refused to deny it to myself any longer.

Oddly, the 'lover' in the scene does not matter. They are often nameless or faceless, and even when it is someone I know and desire, it doesn't make the fantasy any more erotic. However, if a partner teases me in real life about it or presses me down hard on a bed or against a wall, the arousal is as instant as in my old dictionary-definition days. I am sexually submissive, and most of my fantasies do focus on submission and objectification, with this being both the most extreme and consistent of them. The idea of transformation and complete loss of control is just as potent to me now as it was over twenty years ago.

Ruth

Ruth is a heterosexual woman in her late teens or twenties. She has a very high sex drive and considers herself to be a very good lover. She reads erotica regularly and fantasizes when alone, as well as before and during sex.

I have many fantasies, involving many different sexual categories. One of my favourites, possibly because it might be seen as a taboo, is dominating a man who would not seem outwardly submissive. In my fantasy, I use lots of sex toys on him to ease him into the eventual, total domination of penetrating him with a strap-on. Something about a man being in such a vulnerable position makes this my favourite fantasy. I would love to act it out one day with a man who would be totally accepting of my fantasy and could go with it.

Rosie

Rosie is a heterosexual woman in her forties. She has a high sex drive. She fantasizes both when she is alone and during sex. She usually fantasizes about someone she knows, but also sometimes fantasizes about strangers: often black men and women. Her fantasies are varied, and include threesomes, voyeurism, exhibitionism, sex with women and teacher/student scenarios. She sometimes fantasizes about watching her husband being taken by another man.

I have always enjoyed the idea of being taken against my will. Even as a child, I would remember having vague fantasies about being dragged into a cave by a Neanderthal-type strong man. I think Sylvester Stallone may have even featured in one of these childish dreams. What can I say, I was a child of the '80s! I also used to fantasize about being tied up and forced to walk the plank by pirates. There was an erotic thrill to the idea of being taken. My fantasies now often involve being tied up and forced to perform with another woman or man, or both.

My current favourite starts with me being given a voucher

for a place where I can get my own porn movie made, for myself and my husband to watch and enjoy. I arrive at a building and am greeted by a large-breasted black woman whose job it is to prepare me. She sits me in a chair and places my legs in stirrups, and I am given a glass of bubbly while she shaves and oils me. I ask whether I can suck on her breasts, as I am getting increasingly turned on by her touch. She smiles and takes her top off and I suck her large, brown nipples. She then tells me that I need to be measured to see what size cock I can take, and she proceeds to take out a tray of dildos of different sizes, from the very small to the monstrous. Slowly, she inserts them into me, one by one, and we quickly get to the very large ones. When we are ready, she sends me to the costume department, where I am dressed in some kind of tight black-leather harness. I am then brought on 'set'. There is a cameraman and a kind of rounded wooden stool with cuffs at either side. I am told to kneel over the stool with my ass in the air. I am then locked into the cuffs and a ball gag is placed in my mouth and tied tight. I am truly vulnerable now, wondering whether I have done the right thing. I am getting nervous, but also hugely aroused.

A few minutes later, a tall black man and the woman from the prep area arrive. He is spreading lube on his massive cock, and I stare at it in horror. It seems far bigger than the largest dildo that had fit into me. I look at the woman. She is strapping a dildo onto herself. She comes up to me from behind and drives the strap-on deep inside me. It feels wonderful. Then the man takes off my gag and pushes some of his enormous penis into my mouth. He comes inside my mouth just as the woman takes her strap-on out of my behind. They then walk away and I am moaning for more.

They return, but this time the woman is at my mouth and pushes my head to her crotch. I lick her wetness as the man fondles and oils my behind. He slowly pushes himself inside me while inserting an oily finger into my ass. He fills me deeper and deeper and my body is quivering and shaking with the pleasure. He goes faster and deeper as I lap at the woman's warm, wet crotch. My body comes in giant waves of orgasmic pleasure. As I come round, I remember that this has all been filmed. The cameraman is smiling and tells me what a great shoot it was. He quickly edits it as I get washed down and brought another glass of bubbly. I leave with a copy of my very own porn film to watch at home.

I sometimes tell my husband these fantasies, but I mostly keep them to myself. I find that as an Irishwoman, I struggle to allow myself to play out these fantasies in the way I would really like to. My husband and I are starting to experiment more, but I am often overcome by the feeling that I am doing something wrong or abnormal. I wish Irish women would talk to each other about sex more. It's even hard for us to admit to masturbation! Hopefully things are changing.

Ash

Ash is a heterosexual woman in her late teens or twenties. She usually fantasizes about her boyfriend, who she describes as a tall, muscular, hairy 'gentle giant'. She has a high sex drive and considers herself to be an above-average lover.

Something that I have fantasized about but have never spoken of is the idea of my boyfriend using sex toys on me. We have a vibrating cock ring that we use, and it's fantastic. But I've thought about the idea of him using a full-on vibrator and dildo on me, in the type of scene where I would be pinned down, or tied to the bed. He would tease me with the toy and with himself, kissing me all over and touching me down there with the vibrator. He would tease me for a long time, until I was begging for it. Then he would ram the vibrator into me – a really big one. I imagine screaming the walls down, the sensation of a really big dildo inside me and the 'rabbit'-like vibrator on the clitoris all coming together at the same time. I love the idea of being at his mercy and not in control, but having the love for each other to be able to do that.

Naughty at Work

Ms Bovary

Ms Bovary is a heterosexual woman in her late teens or twenties. She has a high sex drive. She is single and mostly fantasizes about a man that she works with who she describes as 'a very fine gentleman'.

I am not the type to have sex in random spots or with complete strangers, but I always get off at the thought of having wild sex in someone else's house – at a party, where no one suspects a thing. In my fantasy, a co-worker and I are at a party in mutual friend's house, and we're both drinking heavily. He keeps glancing over at me throughout the night, his cheeks colouring when we lock eyes. As the night wears on, I end up in the hallway on my own. Suddenly he is standing near me; I can smell his gorgeous cologne. I can see the want in his eyes. We flirt and chat, the tension steadily growing, until he leans in close and whispers into my ear, 'I want to fuck you so badly.' He pushes up against me. I can feel the pressure from his erect penis against me, and my breathing starts to become shallow. I don't want to look up at him. His hand moves down to mine, grabbing it, and he walks me to the bathroom. The minute we lock the door, we start kissing vigorously. His hands move around my body quickly, grabbing my ass and breasts. He lifts me up. We grind against each other, not noticing how much noise we're making as he slams me into the door. Suddenly I'm ripping off my tights. He works away at his belt as he watches me remove my underwear. He clasps my hips, turns me around and pushes me against the sink. I can hear his pants fall to the ground. He pulls up my skirt and groans as he drives it into me, again and again.

Carrie

Carrie is a bisexual woman in her thirties. She has a high sex drive and her most common sexual fantasy is about a particular work colleague. She is married.

I'm at a hotel bar and I see a guy that I work with. Damn he is cute . . . but I'm married. He catches my eye, and I suddenly blush. I'm getting hot, my blood is pumping around my body and I feel a throbbing in my underwear. I want him. He comes over to me.

'Are you here alone?' he asks, in a seductive manner.

'I am', I say.

'I think we should get a room,' he says.

I agree. He smells divine; I want him, my body is craving him. He bangs open the door to the room and we are kissing passionately. He pulls off my clothes and I do the same to his. Oh Lord, what an erection. He pushes me onto the bed. I can't wait for that erection to enter my thumping wet vagina.

Mary

Mary is a heterosexual woman in her thirties. She has a high sex drive and usually fantasizes while she is having sex. She often fantasizes about an old work colleague, but also about her partner and about sex with women.

I arrange to meet a man I used to work with in hotel bar. I am wearing a tight-fitting dress with stockings and suspenders. I am not wearing any knickers. He comes over and kisses me. We have a drink at the bar, and I let his hand slide up my skirt. He realises that I have no underwear on. I notice his cock harden. He leans over and kisses me while his hand rubs me and makes me wet. I begin to throb. We stop and decide to go upstairs to the hotel room. When we get past the door, he kisses me on my lips, down my neck and over my breasts, and then takes my dress off. He strips and throws me onto the bed, turning me over onto all fours. He slides in and out, slowly teasing me over and over till I'm about to explode. As I'm about to cum, he flips me over one last time, so that I can wrap my legs around him while I come hard on his cock. I kneel down and lick his balls, then take his hard cock in my mouth while I rub his balls. I keep sucking and licking and tasting him till he's about to cum. Then he puts it between my breasts and comes all over them.

Angel

Angel is a heterosexual woman in her thirties. She mostly fantasizes when she is alone. She has a high sex drive and is currently single. Her fantasies are normally about a friend of hers who doesn't know that she has feelings for him. She finds his ruggedness and wicked sense of humour very attractive.

There's this guy from work. He has no idea about the filthy, dirty thoughts I have about him, and how I want to be dominated by him. As he's tall and broad and I'm petite, I can just imagine him sweeping me up onto his shoulder and carrying me off to have his wicked way. I imagine being taken away to an old castle, staying in a room with a four-poster bed and fireplace. I'm dressed in black stilettos, fishnets and panties. He ties me to the end of the bed. I'm facing the front, so that I can't see what he's going to do to me. I hear a clap against his skin. He undoes my panties and starts to redden my bum with a leather paddle. The sounds of the slap are such a turn-on. I whisper, 'Harder', and he obliges. My skin tingling, he kisses my neck and starts to play with me between my legs. He can feel that I'm ready, and he is too, and I urge him to untie me and lay me on the bed. I need to have him now, right now, but he has other plans. He gently kisses my stomach, slowly making his way down. Then he stops, taking a glass of champagne and pours it between my legs, for the best tingles ever. I don't want the cool tingling to stop, but I cannot wait for him to have me. I grab his curly brown hair, pulling him up so that he can see what I want. I clench my legs around his waist and whisper, 'Oh my God . . . '

Josephine

Josephine is a heterosexual woman in her forties. She regularly fantasizes about men at work. She works long hours in a male-dominated environment, in a highly stressful job. She usually fantasizes when she is alone and sometimes when she is having sex.

I work with very successful, ambitious men. There's something really attractive about this type of man, even though they sometimes drive me nuts. There is one that I fantasize about quite regularly. He is tall, dark and pretty handsome (cliché, I know). He is funny, though – really funny. That is the final clincher for me: a man who makes me laugh. I find him sexy as hell. He is a bit of a mover and shaker too. I'm sure that he is really well hung and great in the sack. We regularly collaborate on work projects, and I often wonder whether he feels the sexual chemistry that I feel. He has a girlfriend, so I wouldn't go there in real life. But I regularly go there in my head.

In my fantasy, he and I are working late on an important project. Everyone else has gone home, but we have decided to stay till we get the job done. We order pizza and eat while we work. I can see him looking at me admiringly as I quickly get things done. We are bent over a table, examining drawings, standing quite close together. He looks at me, smiling, and says, 'You're pretty good at this, aren't you?' My hair is escaping its ponytail, and my glasses are slipping. I stand up straighter to fix my hair, but before I can respond, he catches my glasses as they fall and hands them to me. I pretend not to notice the spark I feel from his hands as our fingers touch, or the look he is giving me. We both laugh and keep working, but the seeds have been sown – the energy is there, and I know he feels the chemistry that I feel.

As we finish up, he suggests we have a drink to celebrate and reaches for a bottle of champagne in the office fridge, kept for guests on special occasions. I know it's probably not a good idea, but I just can't resist seeing where this might go. We have a drink and toast our success, and as I start to tidy up the desk, I can hear him put down his glass and walk up behind me. He sits down on the chair and gently pulls me onto his knee. I can feel his erection through his suit trousers, and, as he starts to nuzzle my neck, I can feel that lovely warmth begin to flow through my pussy. I know what is going to happen and I am thrilled. I turn around and he looks at me, waiting to see if I am going to slap him or kiss him. I do neither. I get down on my knees and open his fly, releasing his manhood from its cage. I lick him all along the shaft of his penis, taking him in my mouth when I reach the top. He is on fire. He sits in his chair with his head back, enjoying every flick of my tongue. I take off my knickers while I'm down there and stand over him, straddling him. He is thrilled to feel my wet pussy as I slowly sit down on him. He is as hard as a rock, and I can't wait to have him inside me. He rips open my crisp white blouse and the buttons ping all over the office floor. He massages my breasts in his big hands and my nipples are erect, loving the sensation. My heels are still on and that just adds to the naughtiness of it all. He puts his hands up my back and pulls me down onto him, hard. I gasp with the shock of his huge cock inside me, but my body relaxes to bring him in, and he is deep, deep, inside me. He clears his desk (just like in the movies!) with one arm, and throws me onto it. He enters me again, and this time we are both so close to coming that we start slowly, but then he goes for it and we both cum together in an explosive orgasm.

Andrea

Andrea is a heterosexual woman in her fifties. She describes her sex drive as average. She fantasizes about sex with women as well as men, and often fantasizes about men from work.

I work in an office with mostly men: in my department there are five guys and one other woman. Lately, when I masturbate, I have been thinking about these men. In the group, there are two guys in their twenties and the other three are in their forties and fifties. My fantasy takes place on a rainy Friday afternoon. The guys are talking amongst themselves, discussing weekend plans. The young guys talk about the local club and mockingly invite me along. I jokingly reply that I could teach them a thing or two. The young guys say that I couldn't handle them, to which I reply that I would eat them for dinner. The older guys cheer and slag, and I feel the heat developing in my underwear and my pulse quickens.

There is a large meeting room in our department and I jokingly invite the younger guys down there to 'show me what they're made of'. At first they laugh, but the older guys slag them, saying they're all talk. The young guys walk toward the boardroom. I leave my desk and follow them. I walk in behind them and close the door. They both grab at me and roughly fondle my breasts. I moan and rub their cocks through their trousers. They are both rock hard. The younger of the two roughly rips my tights and panties down. He is surprised to see my lack of pubic hair and roughly starts to finger me. I'm so excited that I feel I might come straight away. He bends me over and forces his cock inside me. It goes in with ease.

The other guy seems shocked by what's happening, so I pull him closer and take his pants off. I start to suck his cock, and he pulls my hair as I do it. I feel the other guy stiffen inside me, and I enjoy it even more knowing that he is about to ejaculate. It drives my orgasm on, and we cum almost simultaneously. I keep sucking cock furiously until the other guy comes in my mouth. I feel amazing and the guys are shocked. When I turn around the three older guys are wanking their cocks, saying that they're next. I say no, but allow them to cum on my face one by one.

I'm so excited after writing this that I need to touch myself – I'm aching to cum. If my husband or colleagues read this they would be shocked. I am actually a quiet and reserved type of person.

Brenda

Brenda is a bisexual woman in her late teens or twenties. She usually fantasizes about someone she knows. Her fantasies include sex with both men and women, and she usually fantasizes when she is alone. Her fantasies mostly centre around people in positions of authority: guards, bouncers or her boss. The object of her fantasies currently is a co-worker. He is a dark-haired, bearded, tall, muscular man.

I'm always at least five years younger than the object of my fantasy. In this particular fantasy, I work in a nightclub. I get to work one night and there's no one around except for one bouncer. He's tall and well built – a rugby-player type. I ask him where everyone is, and he just smiles. He walks over and lifts me up onto a table. I'm five-foot-nine, so being lifted is quite the thrill. From there, he kisses my neck and pulls and grabs me, dragging me close to him. Before I know it, we are having sex in a dark corner against the wall of the nightclub. There's something about just the two of us being there and him wanting me so much that turns me on. It's like I'm the most desirable woman in the world at that moment, and we're alone so no one can take that away.

The Great Outdoors

Emma

Emma is a heterosexual woman in her forties. She occasionally reads erotica and has various fantasies, including threesomes, exhibitionism, voyeurism and sex with other women. In her fantasies, her lover is always the boss in the relationship. This story is written as a description for her fantasy man of what she would like to do with him.

It's another beautiful day, the kind we've gotten used to these last few summers. I've a few days' leave from work and have decided to surprise you by showing up unannounced. I pack my bag, ensuring that I don't forget to include a few things I know you'll like. Even doing this starts my heart beating in anticipation of what I imagine is going to happen when we meet. During the drive to your place, I play around with different scenarios in my head. Will I be meek and mild or will I take control? Then again, maybe I'll be both. Nothing like some role reversal! Nearly there now, driving like a bat out of hell or, as you say, 'Mrs Schumacher'. But as I say, there's no harm with a bit of recklessness if there's some control being exerted. The beating in my heart has moved down further to that place that is starting to throb with excitement, as it always does when I think of you.

As I arrive at your driveway, the gates are open, and I continue on up. Your jeep is parked outside. There's a lot of noise coming from the stables: hammering and banging, the loud sounds of metal on metal. You must be erecting the gates to the new stables. I know every thud is you banging with all your might. I see you in my mind's eye, raising and lowering those muscular arms, hairy and strong. It won't be long now till I'm in those arms. I can't wait. I decide there and then that I'm not going to wait.

I get my bag from the car, and outside the locked door, I take my clothes off and eagerly put on black stockings and skimpy briefs, stopping to touch myself. I'm ready for you, all hot and wet, but I can wait because I know you're going to be worth it. I take my hand away and reach for my lacy black bra, brushing my nipples, which are as hard as bullets from the slight breeze and the thought of you sucking them. I quickly pull on a black miniskirt, and a white shirt, tyong it in front so that you can see my cleavage. Lastly, I put on red stilettos and some red lipstick.

I grab the latch and open the door slowly, so as not to surprise you. The noise is deafening but you are oblivious to it as you are wearing ear protectors. You have your back to me, engrossed in the job at hand. You have the gate attached to the railway sleeper on one side and are just fixing the bracket for the bolt to the other sleeper. I'm standing there watching you work – I love to see you getting hot and sweaty. I really admire your strength and stamina. There's no job you can't turn your hand to.

You shut the machinery off. You remove your ear protectors and turn around, not expecting anything out of the ordinary. Well, how about this for a surprise? The ear protectors come clattering to the floor, your mouth opens but no sounds come out. I start to sashay towards you, watching you watching me. You are drinking me in with your eyes, your pupils dilating, getting bigger, just like the bulge in your jeans. You rush towards me and lift me up, covering my lips and neck with hot, breathless kisses while pinching and kneading my ass as you spin around with me.

You begin to speak, but I put my hand across your mouth. I tell you that we can talk later, but, for now, you're going to do as I please. I motion to a corner of the stables where the hay is piled loosely, ready to feed the horses. You bring me over and put me down. You rip my shirt off of me, and I do the same to yours. All the time, we are frantically kissing and touching each other. I unbuckle your belt and pull down your zip. I take you in my hand and feel how hard you are, like a stallion. You remove the rest of your clothes while I continue to stroke you, moving my hand up and down along the shaft the way you like me to. You reach around and unclip my bra (with one hand of course!). Then you bend down and nibble, suck and flick my nipples. You keep doing it because you know how turned on it gets me, and that I feel it between my legs, tingling and throbbing.

You reach down and touch my pussy, now wet and ready. You lay me back onto the hay and spread my legs wide. You just look for a few seconds, and then you get on your knees and then you start licking me, very slowly at first, moving your tongue up and down and round and round. I love the feeling of your tongue on the most intimate part of me. You put your tongue inside me, moving it around. God it feels so damn good, especially as you are squeezing my breasts, the fullness of them in your strong hands, tweaking my nipples between your fingers. You really do push all the right buttons.

I feel your hardness banging against my leg, and I start to stroke you with my instep. At the same time, I feel the sensations mounting in my pussy as you work your magic on me. I am moving slightly now, as you lick me faster. I sink lower into the straw and it scrapes against my skin, something I've never felt before. It's like being stung and scraped at the same time. I like it. I'm almost there now, nearly ready to go over the edge, though I'm going to hang here for a few more seconds, relishing the climb to the climax I know I have to give into.

And then that's it. I call out your name as I cum, moaning and laughing. What a great feeling of release. I bring your mouth up to mine and kiss you long and deep, tasting myself on your lips, tasting what you taste. I start to run my hands over your hairy chest and all over your body, scraping you with my nails. I bury my face in your chest hair, I love how that feels.

I touch your back and butt, light, feathery touches. I scrape the insides of your thighs just the way you like it, and play with your balls, cupping them and scraping them slightly. You are moaning, and start telling me that you can't wait any longer. You grab my hair and pull me up and push me front-facing against some stacked bales. You spread my legs and push my skirt up over my ass. You put your fingers in my pussy, feeling my hotness. You're nibbling and kissing the nape of my neck, running your hands all over me. You slap me on my left ass cheek and, when I shout out, you ram your hard, throbbing cock into me, and in and out you go, faster and faster. All the while you're telling me how good it feels to be deep inside me, how hot and good it feels. I reach behind and grab your ass, going with the rhythm, feeling your big cock as you fuck me hard. Faster and faster, until your moaning gets louder and you shout out my name as you explode inside me. We fall onto the hay and lie there still joined together, and fall asleep, spent but happy.

Cara

Cara is a heterosexual woman in her thirties. She is a stay-at-home mother who does the odd bit of writing. She is married and regularly fantasizes about an extremely sexy six-foot-something guy who she sees jogging near her house during the summer, wearing just a pair of shorts. A common theme in her fantasies would be the strong woman being able to ask for what she wants and gets it – her way. This woman doesn't always let the man take the lead, though sometimes he does, and that's good too.

It's a warm summer's day, and I am in the forest with my boyfriend. We get caught out in a sun shower and have to race back to the car. Luckily, we are parked under a large copse of mature oak trees and this provides a nice umbrella. We are both soaked through and, as I try the handle of the door, I look up to see him staring at me. I glance down to see what has caught his attention.

Due to the good weather, I had opted to wear a sheer summer dress dotted with red and yellow flowers. It is buttoned the whole way down the front, plastered to me and leaving nothing to the imagination. As a nubile twenty-something, I am confident enough not to need underwear. I feel my nipples hardening under his gaze, and he takes a step towards me. I feel something liquid and wet melting between my legs and realise it is pure, sheer unadulterated sexual power and desire.

He is getting closer. I am backed against the car. I can feel the material of my dress sticking to the tops of my thighs. My breath quickens and I lift my chin to meet his gaze. The desire and want reflected there give me a little start. His eyes are black, and his hand reaches out to touch me. He closes the distance between us with a final step, and as his lips come down on mine. His thigh presses between my legs, opening them.

My legs part slightly to receive it, and my mouth opens to his dipping tongue. A small moan escapes me. A little nip on my lower lip breaks our kiss, and he presses his mouth to the side of my neck mumbling how sexy I am. I grin into his shoulder, and I take the lead by opening the buttons on my dress, exposing my breasts to the warmth of the sun and the rain, and then to his lips. The thrill of foreplay out in the open turns me on even more. Anyone could see us.

Then there is the maddening pleasure of his hand going under that dress to find me. I am so hot and ready to receive his touch – his finger deliciously cool against me. He explores me gently, his lips moving over mine and covering my mouth. My eyes fly open as I explode onto his hand. I shudder and buck gently, my thighs tightening around his fingers, trapping him, keeping his thumb there, stroking me. I bite down on his shoulder as his other thumb lazily scratches my exposed nipple, bringing me down from the sheer pleasure of it.

I look up at him. 'Fucking amazing. I want more.' I reach behind me and open the car door. I sit in and lean back a little, my dress sliding down my shoulders. His eyes follow my movements. Then he reaches in and leans over me, his hands opening the rest of the buttons on my dress. It falls open to the waist. I feel alive, sexy, powerful, desired. I am hungry for more. I like the way he is looking at me. I like my inhibition; the strong, innate need to be satisfied. It is a primal urge and I revel in it.

My body, my confidence and my heat tell me to lay back a little more, to bring my legs up and give my thighs a little slack. My dress is gaping at the waist. The warm summer breeze wafting through the window is caressing my nipples, keeping them erect. I sigh and close my eyes, parting my legs just the tiniest bit. I am braless but wearing simple, white cotton panties. After what seems like an eternity, I feel him parting my mouth with the tip of his tongue, using his fingernail to scratch my nipple. It is delicious and sweetly at odds with the gentle probing of his tongue. He bends his head to my unattended nipple. A little suck, a little graze, a little pull. Wet and slippery.

My head falls back and my legs open some more. His hands find my buttocks and pull me down on the seat; hot, wet lips tracing a slow, agonising trail across my stomach, my knees splayed against the seat and the dashboard. I raise my hips and he kisses his way down to my lower stomach, one hand working under the leg of my cotton panties and I feel that fingertip again. I sigh in utter pleasure as my hands grip the seat. I lift my head to see him watching my reaction.

Still holding his gaze, I feel my panties being pulled to one side, exposing me. His hands grasp my buttocks as his head dips between my open thighs and he kisses me, his finger still working. It doesn't take long: soft, wet tongue, probing me gently. Cool finger working. I struggle under his tongue, wanting to lift, to raise, to reach and catch those waves. He holds me still until the last second, and then I soar. Up and up.

I pant – wet, gasping, still not finished. This time it was going to be for real. As he looms in over me again, I grab him, snap open his jeans and pull him onto me so I can trap him. I am still pulsing, still finishing and he grabs my white cotton panties and tears them so he can slide up and into me.

I arch to meet him and climb, hungrily, greedily towards

it, my breath rising again and exhaling in little cries, urging him on, faster, faster, a little harder, more, more, *more*! He groans and falls against me as I relax around him, spent, my hair slick and wet against my forehead, my inner thighs trembling and shaking. We laugh and his mouth finds mine and kisses me hard.

Louise

Louise is a heterosexual woman in her late teens or twenties. Her fantasies normally include men she already knows. Lately she has been fantasizing about a man she met on Tinder.

He's from Wales and he is a farmer. One of my favourite dreams is one where I visit him on his farm and he's showing me around. He takes me to the barn and brushes up against me; I can feel how hard he is. I'm instantly wet and turned on. He turns me around and kisses me hard, lifts up my top and bra to start playing with my nipples. He shows me over to a pile of hay and slowly pushes me down. He grinds on me, teasing me. Finally he pulls down my pants and underwear and goes down on me. I'm so wet. I take off his pants, and he's very erect. I stroke his balls for a minute or so and then he turns me over and enters me from behind. He's thrusting hard and deep while I touch and play with my breasts. The sensations are overwhelming. I moan with pleasure and excitement until we can take no more. We both cum. I continue my tour of the farm.

Lily

Lily is a twenty-seven-year-old heterosexual woman. She is married, and although she usually fantasizes about her partner, she also sometimes fantasizes about sex with other women.

Although I thoroughly enjoyed the *Fifty Shades of Grey* trilogy, my secret fantasy isn't quite as scandalous. I don't believe so, anyway. It's one I haven't thought of in a while. I'm twenty-seven and have been married for just over two years. Maybe I don't think I need to fantasize. Sure, that's what the husband is for. But there is something that I have always wanted to try. My husband is up for it – it's actually me who keeps making excuses.

I imagine a hot summer's day. The clothes we wear are light. We are driving in the countryside in a wide-bonneted, American muscle car, with the roof down. He pulls into a quiet, secluded spot. The fully leafed trees cover us but allow some sunshine through, giving us just enough privacy and just enough vulnerability. I step out of the car and sit against the bonnet. My short, flowy skirt protects my bum from the heat of the engine.

I place my palms on the warm metal surface and lean back. The wind washes over me, cooling me down. It flutters through the trees. Light dances all around us. My loosely tied hair sways in the breeze. He walks around the car to me. He pushes me onto the car and provocatively opens my legs. He steps into the gap and pulls me that bit closer to him. He leaves his hand on the small of my back for just a moment as he stares into my eyes. Our noses are almost touching. I can smell his Hugo Boss aftershave. I feel his excited breath on my lips. He gently pushes my nose aside to give me a soft kiss. He continues to kiss me; his eyes open as his hands begin to wander. They move up from my lower back to my shoulders, around to my bare legs. He slowly brushes against my knickers at my soft spot. He caresses the skin showing between my blouse and my skirt. I start to tingle as his hand reaches up my back to unclip my bra. I feel it pop open. He massages that part of my back, relieving the strain the fabric has caused. He follows this pressure line around to the front of my torso until his finger skims under my breast. My skin tingles all over. The tension inside my body is heightening. I'm breathing hard and lightly scratching his arms and neck.

I break the connection momentarily to pull his T-shirt over his head. I kiss his chest, letting my hands roam and caress every muscle. He unbuttons my blouse just enough to free my breasts and remove my bra. As he cups them, I let out my first moan: a mini release for my body. He squeezes my breasts and rubs each nipple before taking it into his mouth, first one then the other. I pull at his hair with each brush of his tongue. My wet nipples harden even more in the cool breeze. His hands move down between my legs. I kiss and bite his shoulders as he pulls my knickers aside, and starts to gently rub my clitoris. I moan more deeply as he touches me in the most perfect, intimate way. He circles the entrance to my vagina, teasingly. He pushes just the tip of his finger inside as he nibbles on my earlobe.

Desperately, I undo his belt and unbutton his trousers. I pull them down to just below his hips and take his penis out from its hiding place. It's already rock hard, but I tug on him just to see the pleasure on his face. He wraps his hand around my bum and pulls me even closer to him. I lean back slightly more on the bonnet, breasts exposed to the glorious elements as he pushes aside my knickers and enters me. The first penetration instantly sends a thrill right through my body. He grabs my rough ponytail and tugs as he speeds up his thrusts, his thighs slapping against mine. I reach for my clit and rub vigorously, enveloping myself in extra satisfaction. Breathing becomes sharper. Bodies entwine. Limbs hold on tighter. I begin to shudder and, as we both reach orgasm, I fall back onto the car and take his weight, as he lets go and releases all his energy. He lays his head on my breasts, his favourite pillow. I stroke his hair as we regain our breath and then begin to laugh. What a gratifyingly marvellous day.

I have another fantasy. The sun is baking hot, shining down on the garden with its intense heat. There is no tree or shrub to offer shade. No clouds skirt across the sky, and the wind is also missing on this day. I lie on a sun lounger in my sexiest red bikini. Oversized dark sunglasses cover my eyes, and a large straw hat sits on my head. I have a small drinks table propped beside me. It holds a covered bucket of ice, alcohol and a cocktail juice mix: everything a girl needs for a hot day in the sun. I mix all the ingredients together and lie back in my chair. That's when he arrives.

With a lawnmower, he begins cutting the grass. He is topless. His skin glistens in the sun with every push of the machine. His arm and stomach muscles flex. As he turns away from me I watch his back muscles tighten and release. I slide my glasses down my nose slightly to get a better look: dark, tall and handsome – yum.

He makes his way over to my side of the garden. He knows I'm watching. I smirk and push my glasses back up my nose. He stops the lawnmower and strides towards me. He takes an ice cube out of the bucket and slips it into his mouth. It is oh-so-very-hot. I hear it crunch as he bites into it. He straddles me on the sun lounger, placing his legs on either side of my thighs. I sink further into the bed. He takes the glasses from my eyes. He takes another bit of ice from the bucket and places half of it in his mouth. He hesitates at eye level and then slowly melts the ice against my skin. He begins at my throat and gradually moves down my chest, between my breasts and down my stomach. He leaves the ice to melt in my belly button. He kisses me hard with a cold mouth and a deliciously cold tongue. Pulling back one side of my bikini, he teasingly licks my nipple with the tip of his tongue. He takes another ice cube in his mouth and licks my nipple again. I gasp and tense with desire. He leaves the fabric pulled back, keeping my breast exposed as he moves onto my other nipple. This time he removes the ice from his mouth, licks me with his icy tongue and then nips me gently. In the refreshing coolness, my nipples hold their rigidity. Again he leaves the fabric pulled back.

He manoeuvres himself away from me, further down

the sunbed, and unties the bows holding my bikini bottoms together. He gently kisses the spots where the bows were tied, and pulls down the fabric covering my private area. With another block of ice, he outlines my most sensitive spots. First my clitoris, then the exterior surface of my vagina. Setting the ice aside, he bends down. He licks my clit, mixing the sensations of coolness and warmth. I tingle and shiver and moan. I tense and grab his hair and clutch at the sun lounger. He kisses my mound. As he places a finger ever so slowly inside me, he unties his shorts. He rises to let them drop off, as I scrabble to kneel and greet his penis as it stands erect. I take him in my mouth, allowing my tongue to roam and explore.

He pulls me up off the lounger, completely naked in the hot sun, turns me around and directs me back onto the bed. I position myself on all fours, aching for him, tingling in anticipation. He lifts off my hat and sweeps all my hair onto my back. He caresses my spine before firmly taking hold of my hips. He enters me in one gloriously sharp thrust. I groan as he does it again. He begins a steady rhythm and leans over to cup my breasts. He rubs my nipples and breathes hard into my ear. My body shivers as I dig my nails into the sun lounger.

All of a sudden he stops, and pulls me up to a standing position. My bum touches and grinds against his penis. His head looks down over my shoulder as he grasps my breasts with one hand and strokes my clit with the other. His hands are all that hold me up. Turning me around, he lays me down on the grass. He lifts my left leg and places it on his shoulder. Again he takes me. This time I squeal and rip grass out of the ground as my chest heaves in lust and yearning. He grabs my breast one last time as we cry out in orgasm and delirium: a sweet, sweet satisfaction.

Jean Ní B

Jean is a heterosexual woman in her late teens or twenties. She is in a relationship with a garda from rural Ireland. These days, her fantasies normally revolve around him and his uniform.

I'm going out with a garda. I've always had a thing for guards, and as you can imagine, I was pleasantly surprised when I found out what he did for a living (and no we didn't meet in Coppers). I thought that we would have loads of 'close time' when he was in his uniform, but we don't. This drives me to fantasize a lot about us having sex while he is in uniform.

My most common fantasy is that I'm home alone while he's at work on a night shift. He's been really busy and we haven't been intimate in a few weeks – I am literally about to explode if I don't get it. To distract myself, I watch TV, but whatever I'm watching there's a sex scene in it. I text him, telling him I'm horny and need him inside of me, but I don't get an answer. A half an hour later I hear the key in the door and am surprised, as he doesn't usually get home until the morning. He comes into the sitting room and pulls me towards him. Without saying a word he kisses my neck and puts his hand up my top to feel my breasts. My nipples are so hard they could cut glass. He brings me out to the front garden and puts me into the backseat of his squad car. We drive to a remote place, and he tells me to get out and I do what I'm told. He puts the lights and sirens on and gets out of the car. He backs me onto the bonnet and spreads my legs. He then leans down and begins to kiss me and run his hands all over my body while I grind myself against his erection. Before I have the chance to do it, he whips out his penis. He then pulls down my girl boxers and enters me, and we have the most passionate sex on the bonnet of the squad car.

Charlotte

Charlotte is a heterosexual woman in her thirties. She normally fantasizes about being with a strong, dominant male with broad shoulders. He is confident and likes to take control, yet he is sensitive, protective and wants to please. She feels completely safe with him and trusts him entirely. This man in her fantasies is normally her husband.

It's a balmy summer's evening. We are walking together, holding hands, laughing and chatting, enjoying the warm evening. He is in a slightly open shirt, looking gorgeous, and I'm in a light floral summer dress that is shorter than what I normally wear. We wander across the countryside and he leads me through an orchard until we come to a more sheltered spot. He turns to me, smiling. He exudes confidence and makes me feel like the only woman in the world. I feel the energy change. There is an electricity between us. He strokes my cheek and brings my chin to his. He kisses me softly at first, as his other hand moves to my waist. He pulls me towards him and I can feel his intentions against me. He deepens the kiss, and I respond, wanting him to kiss me, wanting him to caress me. His hand moves from my jaw and runs up my back, sending shivers through me. It comes to rest at the base of my neck pulling me further into the kiss. His other hand moves down from my waist to my behind. He massages and kneads my bottom before he parts my legs and starts to fondle me below. He send tingles through me, helped by the open-mouthed kisses that he places down my neck as he makes his way to my breasts. He kisses, squeezes and sucks my nipples and breasts while still working below until my legs feel like jelly. He lies me down on the grass.

I am aching to have him inside of me, to feel the relief of him thrusting deep into me. His mouth returns to mine and he kisses me long and deeply, gently pushing into me. I feel complete. He fills me again and again, thrusting deeper and deeper, almost urgently. We hear voices and pause, holding our breath. My heart is beating loudly. We wait. The voices drift away. We smile and return to our passionate lovemaking until we both peak in pure bliss. Then we lie cuddled together as we wait to return to reality.

Another fantasy I have is to have both my wrists tied to the bed, with a blindfold on. I am dressed in a sexy bodice nightie (which makes the best of my assets) and he is totally in control. He will caress every inch of my body, setting me on fire, and I will be helpless to stop him. In his own time, he penetrates me deeply and slowly. Cupping my face in his hands, he kisses me and thrusts faster and faster, harder and harder. There's nothing I can do but to give myself up to him and enjoy the ravaging.

Sex with the Ex

Suzanna

Suzanna, a lesbian, has a high sex drive and considers herself
to be a very good lover. She fantasizes all the time about a girl
she used to see who was tanned and toned, and had a shaved
head. She describes her as the most delicious creature she has
ever seen.

Her freckled face taunts me in the most innocent manner. I
want to kiss her all the time. I want to stroke her long legs,
put my hand between them and feel her get wet from my
touch. I think I'd play with her clitoris first – she loves to
play. I'd make her squeal and giggle until she moaned for
more. Then I'd gently fuck her until her breathing went into
a slow and steady pace. I'd fuck her harder then, until she

gasped and pleaded for more. I would put myself inside her and wait till she came all over my outstretched arm. Then I would kiss her body all over, licking her pert nipples until her juices flowed over me. I can smell her on me. I inhale. I smell delicious.

Aine

Aine is a heterosexual woman in her forties. She has an average sex drive, and her fantasies usually include her first lover who was a lot older than she was. She lives in rural Ireland and is married.

My husband is wonderful at many things in life, but being my lover is not one of them. He is also only my second lover. My first was an older man I met in my early twenties, a wonderfully sexual man. Sex with him was intense, and we made love at every opportunity, everywhere we could. I knew by the look in his eyes when he was going to take me, and that look alone was enough to make me wet. Every time we had sex we would both orgasm, and more often than not it would be together.

Most of my fantasies involve him and that time in my past, when orgasms were part of daily life. In my favourite fantasy about him, we kiss passionately, licking each other's faces. He undresses me slowly but forcefully, never taking his eyes off me. He cups his big hand over my pubic bone and moves it up and down until I am so wet that his fingers slip inside me. Often he is still dressed from the waist down and I can see the shape of his erect penis pushing outwards.

He takes his clothes off and kneels on the bed, pushing my legs apart, then he rubs the tip of his hard penis against my swollen pussy. I want him, I ask him to put himself inside me. Staring down at me, he grips himself tightly with one hand, pulling his foreskin up and down slowly, squeezing the top between his thumb and his fingers. A clear, pre-cum liquid squirts out, dribbling down his fingers, and he is ready, I am ready. That pre-cum is the 'trigger' in my fantasy; knowing that he is about to enter me, hard and virile and pumping with testosterone. He pushes himself inside me, his teeth clenched, pumping me.

Honore

Honore is a heterosexual woman in her sixties. She lives in rural Ireland. She usually fantasizes about men she has been with in the past. Recently she is fantasizing about a man she was with last year.

We are sitting on a sofa, and I turn and kiss him. I get up and stand in front of him. I press my body against him with my legs on each side of his while I kiss him, making him open his mouth until I want to be swallowed by it. I am getting wetter all the time, and moving up and down his body in quick movements, feeling his hardness. I move my hand down to his chest and softly start to pinch his nipples. Then I unbutton his shirt and really go mad, sucking his nipples, kissing his chest, moaning and slowly unbuttoning his trousers. I undress and get on him again and we move at a faster rhythm. I bring him upstairs and lie on the bed and pull him beside me. We caress each other. He touches the insides of my legs and I sit up on top of him with his penis inside me as I move back and forth. My body leans back, my head and hair touching his feet. I get off and lie sideways so that he can hold my breasts in his hands as I press my bottom into him. His penis is between my legs as I move back and forth rubbing against me as I cum in small orgasms and scream. I change position, lying on my back with my bottom pushed up and get him to stroke me and go on top. I cum again, in a huge orgasm, and collapse onto the bed.

Jane

Jane is a heterosexual woman in her late teens or twenties. She is single. She has a high sex drive and usually fantasizes about a stranger. This stranger is stereotypically tall, dark and handsome. The man never starts off as a full person – initially it might just be the hands – but he emerges as the fantasy develops.

I never felt like I was allowed to feel sexual. This sort of fear is put into women by the threat of assault and rape. It caused me to hide that side of myself for a long time. I hid it until I had an encounter that even remembering now makes my body eager for more.

There was a tentativeness in his body and in mine. We were anxious to see where the night was about to take us, but also scared to let our freaky sides out. He had a full-length mirror in his room. I stared at us reflected in it, his body pressing up against my back. I could feel how hard he was, and felt giddy with life. I let my hand slide back, and felt a shiver of anticipation as I held his very firm penis. He grabbed for me and we slid up against the mirror. He pulled off my dress and ran his hands down my back, grabbing my ass. He pulled me to him and bent me over and entered me. I inhaled, feeling the intake of it all, feeling so alive. He lifted me back up and carried me to the bed. Laying me down, he surveyed my body, running his hands all over me, stopping to remove my bra and kiss my breasts. I arched my back and he manoeuvred down. He began licking and sucking until my whole body was on fire. Then he pulled back to tell me how turned on he was, knowing I was close, he toyed with me. He entered me and pushed in and out, in and out until my body exploded. I felt like all my nerve endings were exposed, and every touch was another climax.

Lou

Lou is a heterosexual woman in her forties. She lives in rural Ireland and used to have a very active sex life. Since she got married and had children she has found that her libido has dwindled. She often fantasizes about ex-lovers, and sometimes about other women. She only fantasizes when she is alone.

I have had many, many lovers over the years. Sex was usually pretty dull. I always loved the flirtation, the chase and the build-up, but the deed itself was often not memorable. There is, however, one particular lover I think about over and over again. He was handsome, funny and clever, and had a great appetite for sex. With him, it was different. I couldn't get enough of him; I still don't know why that was. We were never going to be more than lovers, there was nothing deeper than that, but I didn't care.

He lived down the road from me. I had known him for several years through mutual friends. I never thought I fancied him until one night when we both got drunk in a local bar and had one of those conversations that goes on for hours and is fuelled purely by unexpected sexual tension. We went home together that night and had sloppy drunk sex that I barely remember. The next day though, waking up with heads fuzzy from the alcohol, we started again and didn't stop all day long.

I remember him coming up behind me in the bathroom as I was getting into the shower, standing in front of a full-length mirror. He was taller than me. He only had to stand there for me to get horny. He was rock hard and just pressed himself against me. My whole body just went on fire again, even though I was sore as we had been at it all morning. He put his hands on my breasts and softly massaged them as he kissed my neck and my face. I had never enjoyed being taken from behind, but I knew this time that I badly wanted it. He bent me down gently and lifted up my hips. I can still feel the strength in those arms of his. He entered me slowly, and I was driven crazy with the need to feel him inside me. His thrusting slowly increased in depth and speed, and I came before him with an orgasm so intense that my eyes felt like they were exploding. He came soon after, and we collapsed on the floor. Every muscle in my body ached. We laughed at how we couldn't stop having sex, and then had a hot shower. I have not had sex like that since then. What I wouldn't do for a few hours with him again.

Violet

Violet is a heterosexual woman in her thirties. She is separated, and usually fantasizes about an ex-lover with whom she had wonderful sex. Other women never feature in her fantasies.

My fantasy isn't wild or even really fantastical. What I feel is comfort: wonderful, warm comfort and touching, and some lovely, connected sex (with lovely juicy bits and a nice hard erection). What I fantasize about most of all is knowing that I will not get pregnant. My partner does not have to use a condom, and can ejaculate inside me. Engaging in sex without fear – that's my fantasy.

Current Lovers

Martina

Martina is a heterosexual woman in her thirties. She fantasizes mostly when she is alone. She usually fantasizes about her boyfriend, who she describes as gorgeous and dark-haired, with hazel eyes and a toned body.

I have been asleep on my front, and I'm naked. I wake up to the touch of my lover running his hands up my calves and the backs of my thighs. I feel his hot breath on my ass as he moves higher up my body, gently massaging me awake. He drops hot, wet kisses up my spine as he goes. When he gets to my neck, he sucks gently on a spot he knows drives me crazy. I can feel my clit tingle when he takes my earlobe in his mouth. His hands move around to my chest, lifting me so he can pinch my nipples just hard enough to get me wet, while he leans around to kiss me. When I start to squirm under him, he moves back down my body. He pulls me up by my hips and tastes my arousal, his tongue dipping inside me. He licks up and down my pussy, telling me how good I taste on his tongue and how pretty I am, bared for him like that. He moves under me to my clit, sucking on it while he dips two fingers inside me. I'm getting closer, and he adds another finger to my ass, fucking me until I scream my orgasm.

Before I've even finished coming he has me on my back with my knees over his shoulders and his rock-hard cock inside me, fucking me deeply and using his thumb on my clit. I tell him that it's too much, too intense, I can't cum again so soon, but he just smiles and says, 'I know every inch of you, that was just a taste of how hard you're going to cum for me.' He tells me to pinch my nipples, hard like when he uses his teeth on them. He's getting closer and I can feel another orgasm building. He tells me to take over rubbing my clit. Never missing a beat, he leans back, and rubs his hands along my legs until he gets to my ankles. Wrapping his hand around each one, he pulls them forward, placing a kiss on the arch of each foot. He pushes my legs back and further apart so he can get deeper.

He's fucking me now harder and deeper. He is watching for the moment my orgasm hits me, then lets go and comes with me. I can feel the hot spurts of his release hit me as he groans my name. The world fades away and I'm floating on the power of my orgasm, every inch of my body alive with sensation. As I slowly come back to reality, he releases my legs, gently placing them back on the bed. He leans over and rubs his nose down against mine, kissing me in that soft way that I love. I open my eyes to his smiling face and he says, 'Good morning, beautiful.'

Orla

Orla is a bisexual woman in her late teens or twenties. These days, she usually fantasizes about her current lover. She normally fantasizes when she is alone. She lists exhibitionism, private dancing for a sexual partner, force fantasies and sex with a stranger among the types of fantasies that she enjoys.

I guess you could call my sexual fantasy a little bit of penis envy. Often when I'm having sex with my girlfriend, I imagine I have a big cock that I want to fuck her with – hard. I don't know why, but imagining myself coming as a man really turns me on. I imagine coming on her breasts and on her belly, and then rubbing my cock on her clit as I finish. All the while, in real life, she is pleasuring me, not knowing what I'm thinking. I am a really girly-girl and don't have any other manly tendencies, but I like the thought of having control and imagining my big juicy cock makes me feel like I have power over her.

Pamela

Pamela is a heterosexual woman in her late teens or twenties. She rates herself as a good lover. She regularly reads erotica and has a high sex drive. She always fantasizes when she is alone, and it's usually about someone she is seeing or someone she used to go out with. She never fantasizes about sex with other women. She has a regular fantasy about consoling or congratulating her lover after a match.

After a long day, I near the house, knowing it will be empty, as my boyfriend has a hurling match, which he has been anxious about performing well for. I had decided earlier that day after texting him a good-luck message that, win or lose, I would make him feel like an All-Ireland winner that night. I have ingredients for our favourite meal in the boot of the car, which I quickly unload. Once inside, I start preparing dinner right away, pouring myself a cheeky mid-week glass of wine as I do so. With dinner well underway and a log crackling in the fireplace, I head upstairs to slip into my (and his) favourite lingerie. I dress as I was – jeans, short heeled boots, a purple silk shirt – and have just set the table when I hear his key in the door.

I hold my breath in anticipation, listening for any indications of the match results. His gear bag drops with a thud to the ground and I go to the hallway to meet him. I wordlessly drape my hands around his neck and kiss him deeply before leading him to the dining table. As I pile up his plate he volunteers details about the match, and soon we move our post-match analysis to the couch in front of the fire. When we have exhausted the events of the seventy minutes of play, I kiss him deeply again, and position myself in front of him on the floor. I untie his O'Neill's tracksuit bottoms and take him in my mouth until I feel him relax totally. He rubs my cheek with his hand, thanking me for the lovely meal as I make my way back up his body, straddling him on the couch, massaging his head and tracing my fingers through his hair while he kisses my neck and slowly opens my shirt for access to my breasts. He nibbles on my earlobes, and I moan my satisfaction. He makes short work of my boots and jeans and soon we are in the throes of a passionate sweaty session on the couch, with limbs intertwined, until we collapse exhausted and satisfied.

Samantha

Samantha is a heterosexual woman in her late teens or twenties. She is currently single. She feels that she is a very good lover, and has a very high sex drive. She has many fantasies, including one about a man she has had great sex with on a few occasions, and another about a friend with whom she discusses her fantasies.

In my fantasy, I meet up with this guy. I know him more in a sexual way than an emotional or intellectual way, so this is most likely why I'm able to be so open with him sexually. I'm in a room, standing by the door. I have heels on and sexy lingerie – hold-ups, really flattering stuff. He just stares at me, caught in my gaze. I walk over and straddle him. He's on a couch. Loads of teasing – I make him want me more and more. We move quickly to a bed where he's taking me from behind and digging his nails into my back. He's fucking me really hard and deep and pulling my hair. I scream so loudly that he has to put his hand over my mouth while still thrusting inside me as deep as he possibly can.

I also get ridiculously turned on by watching or making a man masturbate in front of me – the want for him to touch me or be inside me is insane.

Kathryn

Kathryn is a bisexual woman in her forties. She lives in rural Ireland, and is currently in a relationship. She has a high sex drive and considers herself to be an average lover. She has submitted more than one fantasy for this book.

I like the cold. Not the damp, grey cold we get here in Ireland, but a crisp winter's day, with blue sky and glittering frost – and ice. He is tall, with thick, wavy black hair that just meets his collar. His voice is old-school Dublin and, as he says my name, it sounds like music. Then, the sound of the ice as it falls into a glass, the twist of the bottle top, the scent of the rich amber drink, and I know what's coming. He kisses me, and his kisses taste of whiskey, but as his lips move to my neck, I hear the gentle movement of ice in the glass. His fingers trace my shoulder, to my breast, around my nipple, and then the sudden burst of cold as ice replaces his fingers – the burst of cold spreads all over me, tingling, and my body is alive. I'm not the person I was – I am sexy, I am beautiful – and as he traces the contours of my body, each bit of me he touches bursts into life.

He lays me back onto the bed, and the cold of the silk sheets underneath me amplifies the shivers caused by the ice. His kisses move down my body. His mouth is on my breasts, then the ice, then his mouth, then the ice. The sensations run over me; I know what is to come. He pours a drip of the ice-cold whiskey onto my belly and licks it from my skin. I stretch my arms above my head and reach for the iron bedstead. He moves so slowly, but each inch is closer, determined. His fingers run up my legs, so cold. He whispers my name and I hear the strength in his voice, the urgency. He needs me, as I need him – he wants me. I am everything to him, and he is to me.

The windows are open and a cool breeze plays over my skin, but I lie still. He parts my legs and his fingers push deep within my folds. Then the ice touches me there, and the cold is too much, I can't take it – but then the ice is gone and his lips are on me, and the warmth floods me, the heat intense. As I relax, as the pleasure builds, I know it is coming again. He stops, and I hear the sound of the ice in the glass. This time, when he licks me, the ice is in his mouth. He plays it up and over my clit, as his tongue swirls around and his fingers push inside me. Just as my hips rise up, and he knows I'm going to cum, he pushes the ice inside me, and looks up, looks deep into my eyes, as I ride the waves.

I like the cold, as I said; every ice cube I drop into a glass in my everyday life, I can feel, inside me.

Alice

Alice is a heterosexual woman in her thirties. She is in a relationship and has a very high sex drive. She usually fantasizes about her partner. Sex for them is all about connection and mutual pleasure – they are wrapped up in each other.

It's his birthday. I've asked him to come meet me at my house before we go out to the restaurant. I've spent all day getting ready. I've had my hair done, and my skin is soft and smells of my favourite body lotion. I take my time getting dressed, imagining his face when he sees me. It gives me a thrill to picture his eyes roving over me, drinking me in. By the time he arrives, I'm wet with excitement. I buzz him in and wait for him to climb my stairs. I wait in the centre of the room, conscious that my scent will be apparent to him. He sees me, and a devilish smile spreads across his face as he takes in my tight red dress and leopard-print high heels.

I twirl for him and whisper in his ear that my underwear also matches. That appears to be his kryptonite, as he roughly lifts up my dress to my waist then bends me over my bed. Without a word he pulls my knickers to the side and slides his cock deep inside me. He fucks me roughly, brutally, holding me down. I cum repeatedly, feeling his cock rubbing against my G spot and hearing his moans, as he hears and feels me coming. I look down between my legs at his trousers around his ankles and see the muscles in his legs pumping hard while he fucks me. His masculinity turns me on so much. He comes loudly. Still breathing hard, I stand up and fix my underwear. I look him in the eyes and tell him that I am going to enjoy eating dinner while his cum drips through my knickers and slowly down my legs. He smiles, then takes me by the hand and out the door.

Rebecca

Rebecca is a heterosexual woman in her thirties. She has a high sex drive. She enjoys her sexual fantasies when she is alone, and usually fantasizes about someone she knows. She has just started casually dating someone and he is the current object of her fantasies.

My sexual fantasy involves having phone sex while I'm working abroad. I've been away for a few weeks, missing physical contact but enjoying the interim substitute of phone sex. I'm wearing my sexiest lingerie and masturbating as my partner is telling me about where his tongue is and what parts of my body he's touching. I'm soaking-wet and longing for him to be inside me. Then there's a knock at the door. He's outside. He flew over to surprise me. He takes two steps inside and I shut the door, drop his pants and slide his dick straight inside me. The phone sex has made him wet and hard too, so he pins me up against the wall and we both thrust until we cum together.

Bubbles

Bubbles is a heterosexual woman in her thirties. She lives in rural Ireland and has just started a relationship with her plumber, who is the object of her fantasies. She fantasizes mostly when she is alone and likes to fantasize about dancing for her partner, or about dominating or being dominated.

He is my plumber. He is the sexiest guy, and has a huge heart. In my fantasy, he comes into the house as my plumber. His strong brown arms lift me up and take me into the sitting room. He kisses me passionately and places me down on the couch. This is his first time he has lifted up a woman like this, he says, and he tells me it feels amazing. He undresses me, and I undress him. We make passionate love, and it feels fantastic.

Maev

Maev is a heterosexual woman in her fifties. She lives in rural Ireland. She fantasizes about a lifelong friend who is a priest. They have known each other for nearly twenty years. Their relationship is incredibly intimate, but necessarily celibate. She has a very high sex drive and is single. This fantasy is about a dear friend, her best friend for twenty years, the man of her fantasies, her soulmate.

My fantasies of you were lively, but you turned them inside out with your own fantasies, fantasies sharpened to a blazing luminous white light by your unusual self-discipline. The intimacies of VoIP and hangout, of words and images, ravish me and melt you. Separated by oceans, we find new erotic zones and extend our desirous empire. Destiny has set us apart, and we meet but for a few short days each year. We spend the rest of the time talking online, or emailing each other, where we give full rein to our desire. We hold nothing back. The language is the language of sex, the discourse of fertility, the images of spear and womb: my womb, your spear, entering and filling each other; we exchange genders and roles.

Closing my eyes, I feel you with me. It is early in the morning, and we have just woken up. We are naked, which is how we sleep together. You gently pull me towards you and we spoon. Your soft breath on my neck relaxes and arouses me at the same time. We are in a lovely, half-awake, drowsy drifting, and feel no need to talk. Your hand moves to my soft belly. You call it my hara, my womb-space, and you have sometimes been on your knees to venerate it as my life-centre. I quiver. You stroke it as I lie with my eyes closed, enjoying your long sensual fingers on my skin, and the feelings they arouse deep inside me, that seem to warm my body from the inside out. You run your hand along my thigh as I press my bottom tighter into you, to feel your delicious manhood enlarge against my cheeks.

The desire to turn around, straddle you and take you inside me is strong, but I take a deep breath and relax into the moment. Your hands move up to cup my breasts, and gently stroke the nipples. Still not speaking, I turn to face you. I stroke your face as we gaze at each other, and reach up to kiss you. Your mouth opens to welcome my tongue, which explores your own warm, welcoming mouth. We wrap our thighs around each other, and I push my breasts into your chest. Your hands grasp my butt cheeks. I stroke your back, and curve to your bottom: the most delicious, most kissable bottom. We relax from the kiss and gaze at each other while I stroke your beautiful face.

I take control. I place a hand on your shoulder and push you back. I lie on you, my powerful thighs between your slim legs, which you wrap tightly around me. Your awakened manhood presses against the lips of my sacred place, filling it with warmth, and a sense of satisfaction and fulfilment. I feed from your nipples, drinking your life and energy, letting them fill me up. I feel relaxed, content, complete. I draw myself up until I am sitting astride you, your queen. You gaze up at me, your face suffused with love and desire, acknowledging my reign. I lean back, resting against your upright thighs, a queen on her fleshy throne, feeling you move submissively beneath me. I enjoy watching you enjoy my body; it fills me with a sense of power and strength, and I feel incredibly sexy. You run a finger down the middle of my belly, and along the inside of my thigh, and back up again. My whole body feels alive and tingling, loved and cherished in a way that I have never experienced before, even after the best sex.

You give me life, my chaste lover, as I do you. Having the luxury of time on our side, we can explore our bodies slowly, tenderly and erotically. Nothing is expected: the pressure of climax does not impact on us. We come back, tirelessly, to each other's ensouled bodies and each other's souls, and never tire of them. Each time, we enter more deeply into one another. The emotional intimacy we experience is new and novel to both of us, taking us on an adventure we could never have envisaged.

We inhabit separate, very different worlds. We cannot marry. Even the intimacy of full intercourse can never be ours. We will never even live in the same country. Over time, what began as a close platonic friendship has grown and morphed and deepened into something beyond anything we could have imagined. The limits, the boundaries we must live within have served only to highlight the eroticism, the desire, the longing that comes from self-restraint. We have discovered myriad ways of expressing these boundaries, through looks, words, actions and stillness. I could never have imagined anything so fulfilling.

Catherine

Catherine is a lesbian in her late teens or twenties. She normally fantasizes about her partner, or about someone famous. She never fantasizes about sex with men, and includes exhibitionism, voyeurism and threesomes in her list of fantasy subjects.

I'm sitting at my desk, working, and my girlfriend comes in to ask me something. She sits down on my lap and kisses and hugs me. We look at each other and kiss again, forgetting what we were discussing. The more we kiss the harder we embrace, and our grips on each other tighten. I slow down the mood, knowing we are both sufficiently turned on. I kiss and lick her collar bone and shoulder, slowly moving up her neck and across her jawline to her lips. She loves when I do this and moans, moving so that her legs are either side of me. My chest becomes tighter, and our breaths become shorter and louder.

Nobody is home, and we both know we can be as loud and as rough as we like. Not knowing how she will react, I stand up and put her down on the desk. Her head is leaning against the wall and she smiles at me, she moves her hands from around my neck to the top of my head and pushes my head down, slowly, between her legs. I look up at her as I firmly tuck my fingers into the back of her knickers and tights and pull them down over her bum and slowly down her legs.

With my fingers wrapped around her knees, I lift her legs over my shoulders, pulling her vagina towards my face. First I do nothing, firmly rubbing her wet vagina over my mouth and nose. I breathe deeply and inhale her scent, as I run my nails down her back. All she wants is for me to lick her. She pushes my head into her. I grab her ass as I lick her very slowly, but hard. I cup the juices from her opening with my tongue, and stroke them up towards her clit. I do this repeatedly, causing her to sink her fingers into my hair.

She pulls hard each time I reach her clit, letting out breathy sounds. Her body tenses and convulses towards me each time I reach the top of her crack. I quicken my pace until her legs begin to shake. Her mouth is pointed at the ceiling as she screams for me to go and faster. Her shaking thighs wrap around my head and push me so hard against her that I'm finding it difficult to move my head or breathe. But I keep going until she lets out a final, orgasmic, high-pitched noise. Her body goes limp, and her breathing slows.

I wipe her juices from my face up and down her thighs, to show her how wet she was.

We get up and fall onto the bed. After giving her such amazing head, my body is ready. My underwear is uncomfortable, and I pull the fabric away from the swollen wet patch beneath my jeans. She sees this and smiles, still in a post-orgasmic daze. We kiss again and she climbs on top of me, straddling me, grinding her pelvic bones against mine. This feels nice, but I want a deeper feeling. I roll her off and look under the bed. After finding what I was looking for I take off all my clothes, watching her limp body, legs slightly spread.

I'm holding a long, smooth silicone shape, curved at both ends. Her end, the penetrating end, is longer and straight just until the tip. My end is shorter but thicker, and fits into me in such a way that I can hold it there. She looks at me. I am standing naked at the foot of the bed with her end protruding out of me, angled upwards. She crawls towards me, and we meet in the centre of the bed. First we kiss. Then I push her away and arrange her so she lies on the bed, face down. Positioning myself directly behind her, I pull her by the hips so that her ass meets my toy.

Her head is still on the bed and I take a second to look at her. Enjoying my position of power, all the while knowing she loves to be moved about. I reach around and touch her clit, still dripping with excitement. My other hand is holding the toy and I slowly wiggle it into place, pushing it into her vagina until it stops. We both moan. My end is pushing into me firmly and her end is pushing into her, upwards into her G spot. I clench my end and pull out really, really slowly, telling her to touch herself. When I thrust into her a second time I do it quicker and harder. The combination of our wet flesh makes a slapping sound. I do it again and again. It feels amazing and she is screaming with pleasure. I am attempting to breathe slowly, trying to delay my orgasm. I turn her over and we fuck harder. This time the toy is vibrating, and each time our bodies cum together it pulsates against our clits, all the while penetrating. We grab onto each other hard. Nails and fingers and teeth are out. Biting and scratching to compliment the intense internal pleasure. We go faster and faster and harder, until we scream and we both cum hard together.

She pushes me off her and the toy jumps out of me, still vibrating. She shoves it in and out of me as I lie on my back. I'm coming and squirting all over her hands and thighs as she kneels over me. It finally stops and we lie together, limp in the puddle, until we fall asleep.

Elaine

Elaine is a heterosexual woman in her late teens or twenties. She lives in rural Ireland. She normally fantasizes when she is alone. She fantasizes about strangers as well as people she knows. These days she often fantasizes about a tall, bearded man with a lumberjack look.

I'm at the kitchen sink doing some dishes and my partner is outside, coming in. He has been out all day working with his hands and he is a bit dirty and scruffy; he still has some dust in his beard. He sees me watching him and he smiles under that rugged beard. I bite my top lip because he knows that beard drives me insane. He strolls into the kitchen all cocky and slowly walks over to where I am. He puts his hands into the sink to wash them, all the while pressed against me. But I'm trapped between him and the sink. I can't move any-where. He begins to kiss my neck, I turn to him and he is now pulling down my pants and sticking his big fingers inside of me. I'm wet with just the slightest touch from him. I moan with delight. He turns me and bends me over the counter, forcing himself inside me as I moan. He grabs my hair with one hand, while his other is on my back. He pounds me as we both grunt and moan.

Rose

Rose is a heterosexual woman in her late teens or twenties. Her relationship situation is complicated. She has a high sex drive and regularly fantasizes about a man she has started seeing.

This is the fantasy I have most often. It's in the middle of the night and my partner and I are sound asleep, spooning in bed. He gently wakes me from my deep sleep, rubbing up against me, wanting me. I can feel his rock-hard erection against my silk nightdress. I'm instantly awake and aroused. It's pitch-black in the bedroom. I start to push back against him, letting him know that I'm awake. Without a sound or a word spoken between us, he begins to touch and caress me, gently at first, his hands running over my breasts and kissing my neck. My nipples are erect and I have such a longing for him.

He begins to run his hands down my body and slowly tugs my silk nightdress up around my hips, exposing me. Still we are not saying a word to each other in the pitch darkness of the bedroom. He runs his fingers over my pussy, feeling how wet I've become. I rub myself more against him, dying for him to enter me. He slips his cock inside me and holds it there for a few seconds, relishing the feeling. I feel so full. Then he starts moving in and out of me, holding onto my hips as I touch myself, faster and faster, until we both explode together. He pulls out of me, and I feel his cum running between my thighs. We fall back asleep instantly, tangled up in each other.

Don't Get Caught

Rachel

Rachel is a heterosexual woman in her forties. She enjoys fantasizing about sex with strangers in public places. Her fantasies are very different to her reality.

I am in an old library searching for something, and I'm in an aisle between two very tall bookshelves. It's very quiet. I don't think that there's anybody around. It is summertime and everyone is outdoors enjoying the weather, but I need to finish this project so I'm stuck in the library. I'm standing on my tiptoes, reaching up to take a book down off a high shelf. I'm wearing a very short skirt that rides up a bit as I stretch. Next thing, I'm aware that someone is behind me; I get the sensation of a presence. I can hear breathing, and I get a very faint scent of maleness – an aroma that isn't unpleasant, but is unmistakeably masculine. All of a sudden, I realise that he's stepping closer to me, so close that he is touching my back, and that's when I feel the hardness of his erection against me. I'm tempted to turn around, but before I can do so, I feel him wrapping his arms around me – one hand on my breast and the other grazing my thigh. He's gentle, but at the same time I can feel his strength, and I know that there's no point resisting, even if I wanted to. I feel his hand reaching up under my skirt, slowly, as if he has all the time in the world. I can feel myself getting wet with arousal. His other hand caresses my breast, and my nipple is standing to attention. Then he moves to the other breast.

Not a word has been spoken, but the air is electric between us, and our breathing becomes heavier, more ragged. As his lips start to nuzzle my neck, I feel a moan building up in my throat, but he hushes me and I know that I need to remain silent. There may not be anyone in the library, but I'm not sure, and the thought of being found in this compromising position is arousing me even more. He has been touching my thighs, teasing me for a while now, and I'm starting to wish that he'd reach higher. I try to reach behind to feel his body, but he won't let me. I'm at his mercy.

By now he has managed to find his way underneath my thin blouse and bra, so that his hand is on my bare breasts, and he starts to become rougher and more urgent in his actions. I long for him to turn me around so that he can suck them, but I also know somehow that if I saw his face it would break the spell. I feel the sensation of flesh against my leg and realise that his bare hard erection is pushing up under my skirt. I want him to enter me so that I can feel his heat and his long hard length inside me. Next thing, though, he pulls my pants to one side and he starts to massage my clitoris, while his cock presses against my anus.

I'm a bit taken aback at first, but then realise that I like the sensation. He has me braced against the shelves, facing the books. He starts using his fingers to take the wetness from my pussy and rub it on my anus and his cock. I've never experienced this before – I realise that I want more. I can't help myself; I start to moan. Now that he has released my hands, I move them down to play with my own nipples and clitoris, helping him out.

Next, he puts two fingers up my cunt, and his other hand is playing with my virginal anus. He gradually inserts a finger. I really like the sensation: it's like being taken by two men at the same time. He must take my submission for permission, because now he carefully removes his finger and replaces it, gently, a little bit at a time, with his cock. I've never had a cock up my arse before and I never thought that I would like it, but this feels so good. He's using his hands to tweak my nipples, harder now and insistent, while he's starting to rock inside me.

I feel so full with his huge member up my back passage, but it's a good sensation. As he rams harder into me, pushing me against the stacks of books, I help out by rubbing my own clitoris. We're both panting now, moving together in rhythm. I feel that I'm about to cum, screaming. I can sense that he's almost there too. As the waves of sensation come over me, I can feel him ejaculating. It's the best orgasm of my life, the sense of relief as I cum is amazing, and the aftershocks just keep on coming, longer than any orgasm I've ever experienced before.

Then, before I can turn around, he pulls out of me, zips himself back up and walks away down the long aisle of shelving. I take a moment to gather my breath and, still dripping with his cum, turn around, but he has vanished.

Triona

Triona is a heterosexual woman in her thirties. She has a high sex drive. She sometimes reads erotica and considers herself to be a good lover. The object of her fantasy can be a stranger or her partner, but if it is a stranger, there is still a sense that she knows and cares about him.

I've just recently entered a new relationship and it is amazing – he makes me feel so comfortable in my own skin that I can tell him my fantasies and explore a part of myself that I probably hid too much in the past. Unfortunately, we live too far apart to see each other as often as we'd like. To make up for that, we like to send suggestive texts and, in my case, drawn-out fantasies that I send in bits, so that we both get hot and bothered at the same time even though we are far apart. He suggested I send this one in, as it is his current favourite.

I'm walking down a street, and my boyfriend is secretly following behind me, waiting to surprise me. I step into this dark building. He comes inside and is pleasantly surprised that it's actually a cosy library, with shelves full of books on all sides, leading up to high ceilings. Everything is dark and richly coloured, and there seem to be several rooms separated by tall doorways framed with heavy curtains. I know that I'm moving ahead, but I can see him move slowly to stay hidden as he makes his way into the depths of the room.

In the background, I notice that there is faint music coming from somewhere. My boyfriend starts moving towards it. There's a light, slightly spicy smell in the air, a little like incense. For some reason it makes the whole situation seem very erotic. As we move through the different rooms, I begin to notice paintings on the walls and sculptures on the side tables that all seem to be very suggestive. There is an image of ladies in a pool, in various states of undress, who at first glance seem to be touching each other sexually, but on closer inspection are only innocently splashing around. From behind one of the sculptures looks like a threesome, with the man thrusting into one woman from behind while she grinds into a woman lying beneath her – but from the front, it's merely an oddly shaped tree.

My boyfriend keeps moving, desperate now to find me, as he feels his body responding strongly to all the stimuli, his gigantic cock strains against his jeans and his sensitive nipples rub against his thin shirt. I feel my skin almost tingling with anticipation. Just then, he turns a corner and sees me. I'm engrossed in a book in the corner of the back room, where he can see that we'd have total privacy to be naughty. He waits a few minutes in the shadows, just watching me, wondering what I'm thinking and why I'm so focused on the book in my hand. He can see that my mouth is slightly open and that I'm biting my lip. My hand is resting on my collarbone, playing with the necklace hanging there.

Just as he is about to make himself known, I slowly move my hand, and lightly run my fingers over the nipple of my left breast. It happens so quickly that he isn't sure if he saw right, but then I look around and start to unbutton the front of my dress, just enough so that I can slip my hand inside of my shirt and cup my breast. Still reading from the book, I take my hand out to suck on each finger before reaching back in to play with my nipple. He has to control his breathing so that I won't know that he is there, as he wants to see what will happen next. I spend a few seconds in that position and I'm beginning to sway on my toes, as if my body could hear the music. I take my hand away from my breasts and slowly move down, pulling the bottom of my dress up at the same time. With a deep sigh, I start to touch myself, slowly and carefully at first.

I am still afraid I'll get caught, but I soon start getting carried away, leaning into my hand while my hips move desperately. I look around, and spot an old upholstered chair stuffed between the shelves. I fling myself into it so I can arch my back up. The chair happens to be pointing towards him, but I don't see him because I'm too distracted. He can see my bare legs, leading up to my wet pussy with my fingers rubbing in circles, dipping in and out, making me moan. He watches as an orgasm slowly begins to build, but can see that I'm getting frustrated because my fingers keep slipping – I'm almost too wet. He slowly emerges from the shadows, making the floorboards creak so I will look up and see him.

At first I get a fright as his face is still in shadow and I don't know it's him. I quickly start to cover up, but then I see him. Although my heart was already beating hard, it goes up another level as I see how turned on he is. Seeing my eyes transfixed by his crotch, he slowly starts unbuttoning his pants, without saying a word or taking his eyes off my face. He keeps moving towards me, removing all his clothes, so that by the time he is right in front of me he is completely naked, and I can hardly breathe at the sight. I try to reach up and pull him down, as I know that having him inside me is all I need, but he doesn't let me. Instead, he sinks to his knees, separates my legs and, after staring deep into my eyes for a never-ending second, he lowers his mouth and starts licking and flicking my clitoris with his tongue.

I can't help but moan out loud and push my pelvis up, so he takes his finger and plunges it deep inside me working in rhythm with his mouth. Almost straight away, he brings me right to the edge and I can't take anymore – I call his name and pull him up. He is very close now too, and doesn't stop me when I wrap my legs around his waist and pull him towards me. We don't play around and, in one big thrust, he pushes inside me, making us both gasp and look at each other. We are still for a split second and then the passion takes over, as we desperately kiss and run our hands over the other's bodies. We move together, sometimes aggressively and sometimes slowing right down to pull back and keep going.

He lifts me, putting his hands around my ass, carrying me to the nearest shelf and leaning me against it. I put my hands above my head for support while he starts sucking my breasts. Both of our bodies are on fire; I can feel him throb inside of me. As we feel the build-up starting again, he lays me on the floor. I wrap my legs around his neck as he starts to fuck me hard. We are both making a lot of noise but neither of us care – all we can feel is each other. I can't believe how big he is, and I seem to be getting tighter around him. I can see his eyes watching me move beneath him, and it turns me on even more so that I'm dripping all over him. My orgasm comes quickly and intensely, and its ripples push him to move faster and harder. With a final moan he comes deep inside of me. We collapse, covered in sweat and holding onto each other while we try to get our breath back.

He is still inside me when we hear the front door open. We wait a minute to see if whoever it is will go away, but then we hear footsteps moving towards us. I'm still wearing my dress so I quickly roll out from under him, button up my front and fix my hair. I leave him rushing to get dressed and meet what turns out to be a staff member, who had stepped out for a chat with a friend. I distract her outside the room by asking about an obscure author. He comes out to join us, slightly flushed and dishevelled, but dressed. We make eye contact, and with a conspiratorial wink I subtly try to draw his attention to my legs. He's confused at first, as I seem to have my legs tightly crossed, but then he sees the faint white line slowly dripping down my thigh, and under-standing dawns. He turns slightly, letting me see my panties sticking out of his jacket pocket. He closes the conversation and moves us outside, where we immediately check into a nearby hotel and have sex several more times before dinner.

For me, setting the scene is as important as the fantasy sex – it creates a real build-up of sexual tension.

Daisy

Daisy is a heterosexual woman in her late teens or twenties. She has a very high sex drive. She usually fantasizes about her partner while she is alone. She met her partner on a drunken night out. He is a lot older than she is, and being with him has made her realise that there is nothing better than a 'manly man' who knows exactly what he wants and how to treat a woman.

I've experienced some of my fantasies in reality, but there are still a select few out there that I am dying to try out. I've been with my partner for a year now, and he is significantly older than me, with a lot more experience. However, I am the one with the explosive sex drive that keeps him on his toes.

My first sexual fantasy is one where we are at a family dinner, and my parents are in the living room, being hosts to the rest of the guests. As I look at my gorgeous guy oozing sexiness, with his witty jokes and smile that melts my heart, I can't help but stare at his crotch. I bite my lip as I take in his rock-hard ass. I feel the need to grab it and thrust into him, pelvises together. With all this sexual tension, I make eyes at him until he follows me out to the kitchen. I take him through into the utility room and pull him against me, kissing, breathing heavily – the excitement of knowing that the family could walk in at any point is just so hot. He lifts up my skirt (I have no panties on) and sets me on the counter. He holds onto my bare ass and uses it to thrust into me, hard and deep. The fear of getting caught is the biggest turn-on ever.

The second fantasy is of my partner being cross and authoritative, and giving me a warning – not in a creepy sadistic way, just being playfully masterful. He bends me, naked, over his knee and gives me a spanking, and then takes me to the bedroom and enters me from behind. I love the feeling of his balls banging against me as he thrusts, of him kissing the back of my neck and gently blowing in my ear and giving my ass cheeky slaps every now and then.

Heidi

Heidi is a heterosexual woman in her thirties. She lives in rural Ireland and is separated. She has a very high sex drive. The person she fantasizes about the most is an ex-partner with whom she shared a lot of fantasies. She and her ex-partner were quite adventurous, and tried some of them out.

I have many fantasies, but I shall share my current favourite. I travel a lot with work, so I regularly find myself passing through the airport. On this particular trip, I have had a big night the previous night, with some of our European distributors, and I am mildly hungover. This generally results in me being very horny; I just get a craving for sex. I have messaged my partner to tell him to meet me. He knows how I am feeling. He finds me in arrivals, in Terminal One. He has come straight from work and is in his suit, his tie hanging loosely round his neck. He hasn't shaved that morning and looks slightly dishevelled, but in such a sexy way. I am wearing a smart navy dress which stops just above the knee. Underneath, I am wearing hold-up stockings, high heels and my favourite sexy underwear: a sheer black bra and knickers. He grins when he sees me, and I feel my face flush. I have been looking forward to seeing him since I got on the plane. I greet him with smile and a chaste kiss. He slips his arm around me and we make our way up to the short-stay car park. He has parked in the corner of the upper floor.

He tightens his grip as we approach the car, my heart thumping. His touch and the closeness of my body to his is driving me wild. I free myself from his grip as I walk between his car and the next. He is still right behind me. I turn to face him and he presses his body up against mine, pushing me back against the car. We look straight into each other's eyes, and I lean in to kiss him. The kiss is ferocious and hard. He reaches down and lifts the hem of my dress, running his hands over the flesh between my stockings and my knickers, and lets out a small, appreciative gasp. I can feel my own wetness, I am positively throbbing in anticipation of his touch.

There are cars driving round, looking for places to park. I snap out of it.

'Come on, open the car so we can get home,' I say, smiling. He opens the car and I open the back door. He is still right behind me, caressing my ass through my dress. I bend over to put my case in the back seat. He lifts the hem of my dress again, slipping his fingers under my knickers to caress my bare ass. I literally tingle all over. I push back against him and stand up, still facing the car. He presses up against me and kisses my neck as he slips his fingers around to the front of my knickers. Then he pulls them aside and strokes me. He tells me he doesn't think he can wait until we get home. He has one hand in my knickers and, with the other, I hear him open his belt and undo his zip.

There are still cars driving around, and the only thing between us and them is the rear passenger door, but somehow they seem farther away now. He is still nuzzling my neck and caressing me. I am already close to coming. This is so crazy, but so what, I want it. I push back against him, daring him to finish what he has started. He spins me round to face him again. We kiss, more gently this time, he is teasing me. I am so aroused that I think I might burst. I position one foot on the rear wheel, opening myself up, inviting him in. In a swift movement, he is inside me. I take a sharp breath. *Oh my God, yes.*

'Harder, faster,' I whisper. My orgasm comes in a blinding flash of light. I stifle a moan, acutely aware that there are other people in the vicinity. He holds me close as my knees begin to tremble, gently sliding out of me.

Once I have regained my composure slightly, he pulls down my dress and refastens his trousers. He grins a wicked grin and slaps me on the ass and says 'Come on, let's get you home so we can finish this properly.'

Grainne

Grainne, who is bisexual, currently has a female lover. They share their fantasies, and fantasize together while having sex. Her sexual fantasies include private dancing for a sexual partner, threesomes, domination and being watched while masturbating.

Right now, my fantasy is surprising my lover at work. Everyone else has left the office. As I lock the door, she's dressed in a fitted black suit with a white shirt. I'm wearing a beautiful dress, stockings, red high heels and my lovely black leather harness and cock. She doesn't see this under my dress – yet. My lover is thrilled to see me, but nervous that her colleagues might come back. I don't say a word. I push her against the wall, kiss her deeply and slowly begin to undo her clothing. I undo her buttons, and delight in her lacy purple bra. I kiss her gently and signal to her to unbuckle her belt, which she does. I'm excited to see if she's wearing the knickers I instructed her to wear: soft lace, perfectly stretched across her mound. She is. I peel down her pants and kneel before her to inhale her scent, kiss her through the lace and kiss her inner thighs. I tease her, my tongue against her knickers. She is craving my touch, craving skin on skin. I gently slide a finger along the edge and, underneath, into her wetness. She's drenched with desire. I motion for her to turn away and bend over her desk. Her pants are around her ankles, restricting her movement. Slowly I caress her fine arse, I kiss her cheeks, slide the cloth across and, kneeling down, I kiss her very wet cunt. She moans deeply; her taste intoxicates me.

Standing up, I lift my dress and let her feel my cock press against her arse. She's a little scared, but so turned on that she gives no resistance. I tease her with the tip while I stroke her clitoris with my fingers. I delight in slowly entering her, allowing her cunt time to open, to permit me to push deeper – to fill her. Her hips push back against me. She begs me to fuck her, and I do, gently, firmly, stroking her all the time. Reaching forward, I free her beautiful breasts and squeeze her nipples – hard. She wants me to squeeze harder. I am incredibly turned on.

I place her on her knees in front of me and tell her to suck my cock, and to gaze into my eyes as she does so. She's very obedient, willing to pleasure me in any way I ask. I lean back against the desk so that she can reach my wet cunt with her fingers between the straps of my harness. She pushes deep into me, filling me, fucking me hard and fast, her mouth on mine. It's so delicious. My fingers find her clit and, as I stroke her firmly, we finally explode, our bodies bucking with the power of our mutual orgasm. Wave after wave rocks us. It's bliss: pure, free and powerful.

Slowly it subsides, and we reluctantly withdraw from each other. We slide off the desk to the rug, and hold each other in the beautiful afterglow. We still haven't spoken. I kiss her softly, pull up her knickers and pants and re-button her shirt. I whisper in her ear that I love her and, fixing my dress, I leave.

Joanne

Joanne is a heterosexual woman in her late teens or twenties. She has a high sex drive. She fantasizes about the different people. Sometimes it's a celebrity, or a man that she's dating or an ex -lover.

I have a fantasy about being on holidays alone (I suppose so that there's no judgement and no one knows me) and meeting a complete stranger in a nightclub. I am dirty dancing with them and riding them in the toilets there and then. I have a real obsession with doing things like that, in places where I could possibly get caught. I love the idea of people queuing outside the toilet, and me inside with a stranger getting my rocks off. I have been known to drag unsuspecting men into the toilets in pubs and clubs, but it has never escalated to full sex, just to oral.

Janette

Janette is a heterosexual woman in her thirties. She has a low sex drive but considers herself to be a good lover. She only ever fantasizes when she is alone, and often fantasizes about sex with other women.

I kept starting this questionnaire and finding myself unable to complete it. The idea of sharing my fantasies was exciting and a bit risqué, but when I actually sat down to write it, I would just chicken out. Why is it so hard? Anyway, here goes.

I have been reading recently about something called dogging. Apparently couples go to car parks, have sex in their cars and let people watch. I was intrigued and a bit disgusted. I looked it up online and realised that it happens all over the country! I would never, ever go do it, and when I told my husband about it he told me that he thinks it's all a bit weird.

I can't help thinking about it though, and it has become a common feature in my fantasies. I don't fantasize when I'm having sex, it's usually when I'm in bed by myself. My dogging fantasies don't really include me, I'm always just watching; I'm one of the pervy people looking into a car with a hot and sweaty couple having sex.

The windows are all fogged up. The woman is beautiful, with long hair, full breasts and gorgeous skin. She's always in the missionary position, and completely naked. The boot door is often open, and he is standing on the ground, shagging her as she lies on the floor of the boot. He is partially dressed, with his trousers around his knees. There are men standing all around the car, masturbating as they watch. I have no idea if this is what it's really like, but the thought of it does it for me.

Woman to Woman

Sheena

Sheena is a heterosexual woman in her forties. She has a high sex drive. She fantasizes when she is alone as well as when she is having sex with her husband. She currently fantasizes about a long-term female friend and an artistic older man she knows.

I have two main or regular scenarios that appear in my fantasies. This one features my female friend. We have a long, subtle and deep friendship, yet we both take care not to spend too much time together. Our lives are very different, and we keep them separate, yet they are and always will be entwined, and we take care to monitor each other from a distance. We had a brief encounter many years ago now and it is this remembered desire and promise that I return to again and again, with both relief and regret for its non-fulfilment.

I imagine her coming over for the evening. We drink a little wine, have some good food and talk about the people we love and have loved. We listen to the music of our youth and we dance a little. We are alone, in her house, and we know we will not be disturbed, as we almost were that first time. Like our first time, it is not a contrived situation. She is far more sexually adventurous than me and always has been, with a predatory streak that attracts and repels me in equal measure. She approaches me slowly and deliberately. She first touches my mouth with her thumb, gently tracing the shape of it, then softly parting my lips. I allow myself to open to her, and I suck her thumb. Then she places another finger inside my mouth, and I suck that too. She moans gently and puts her other hand on my breast, and pinches my nipple hard. I suck harder, and she takes her fingers out of my mouth and slips them between my legs, firmly cupping me.

I am wearing a skirt and tight silky knickers, and I can feel the intense heat of her hand. I push against it, and she strokes my clit with her finger; it is sensitive and swollen already, and the crotch of my pants is wet. She comes up behind me and, still firmly stroking me, bites my neck and whispers in my ear. She tells me how she likes that I am so wet for her. She slips a finger inside me, tells me she wants to taste me, that she's wanted that for a long time. She tells me that she wants to fuck me with her tongue, with her mouth. Would I like that? Do I want that? She tells me to tell her what I want. All the time she is fingering me and pinching and pulling my nipples, rubbing her palm over them.

I am shaking by now, and I want her hands on me, her fingers in me, her mouth on me. Turning around to her, I push her shoulders down. I tell her I want her mouth on me. I tell her that I want her on her knees, that I want her tongue, that I want her sucking me, sucking my cunt and licking me. I want to cum on her face, in her mouth. I want her to fuck me with her tongue. I tell her how I've wanted that for a long time.

She kneels and opens her mouth on me. She kisses me like my cunt is my mouth and she pushes her tongue inside me. It feels so unbelievably good, like she is kissing the very heart of me. She keeps her eyes open. I love the sight of her looking up at me, her head between my legs, her face shining with my juices and her voice huskily murmuring her pleasure and mine.

I am touching myself as I imagine all of this and by now I am on my knees, arching and rubbing myself. I orgasm fast and hard, and fall back on the bed, wondering what might have happened had I let her have me that time, and wishing that I had.

Amber

Amber is a heterosexual woman in her forties. She has a high sex drive and considers herself to be a good lover. She has sexual fantasies about her husband, as well as about strangers. She also has a recurring fantasy about a faceless woman.

Before ever having sex, when all I knew was that masturbating felt good, I used to fantasize about creating some kind of masturbation machine that could bring me to orgasm over and over again. I pictured myself just lying there, letting the machine do the work, and getting off without stopping. It seemed like something out of a Frankenstein movie, with metal contraptions – not necessarily the most comfortable machine. I've since been to the Sex Museum in New York City, and realised that there are many of these 'contraptions' out there. The 'Rabbit' that featured on *Sex and the City* was my eye opener to the world of vibrators, and seemed like a more realistic and discreet answer to my fantasy.

While my only foray into homosexuality was as a young-ster, with my friends, when we practiced kissing each other and the like, I've always fantasized about having oral sex with a woman – receiving it and giving it. I picture kissing a woman, having her suck on my nipples, taking them in her mouth and licking around their most tender parts, then slowly making her way down to the apex of my thighs, where she licks and sucks my clitoris, bringing me to a mas-sive orgasm, all the while pinching my nipples.

I also imagine reciprocating, feeling her body writhe against my tongue, my mouth giving her pleasure, hearing her as she explodes. I must admit I feel rather guilty, but this is often the image I have in my mind as my husband brings me to orgasm. It's rather difficult for anybody other than me to bring me to orgasm, and I find this scenario helps me to get really aroused and achieve climax. Not sure what the sex therapist would say to that.

Anna

Anna is a heterosexual woman in her forties. She lives in rural Ireland. She considers herself to be an average lover, and has an average sex drive. She mostly fantasizes when she is alone.

In my fantasy, I see another woman (a stranger) making love to my husband. I'm hiding, so only my husband knows that I'm watching. She performs oral sex on him, and lets him cum all over her breasts. I want to enter the room and rub it into her breasts like a lotion, but I can't. I'm heterosexual, but something makes me want to suck her nipples and taste her down below, just this once. I suppose it's curiosity, as my husband always spends ages going down on me.

Lisa

Lisa is a heterosexual woman in her late teens or twenties. She lives in rural Ireland. She has a very high sex drive, and regularly reads erotica. She is single, and often fantasizes about having sex with a policeman and dominating him.

One fantasy I have is about a female eye specialist – it's the bi-curious part of me. I walk into the exam room for eye tests and, standing before me, is a female optician. She has long, wavy blonde hair that ends close to her bra line. Her face is of movie star quality. She knows she radiates beauty, but she is still demure. Her body is toned, with curves in the right places. Under her white work coat (which is open) she wears a knee-length skirt with a camisole, and small kitten heels. Her breasts strain gently against her top. I can tell that she is wearing stockings and suspenders when she crosses and uncrosses her legs.

She begins with the usual eye examination, then tells me she wants me to watch a short movie clip so that she can study my eye movements. This is where it gets unusual. As the clip begins to play, she walks over and stands behind me, moves my hair over to one side and begins to slowly caress the nape of my neck. It sends chills down my spine – it certainly isn't what I was expecting during an eye examination. As she continues to gently caress my neck, I can feel her breath on my naked flesh. My mind goes into overdrive, thinking this shouldn't be happening, but there is a pull that I can't resist.

As her lips start to move along my neck I shiver in anticipation, wondering what will come of it all. She slowly moves around my neck to my lips and begins to kiss me softly. Her kisses become more urgent and animal-like, her hands roaming and searching my body, seeking a reaction. I begin to lose control and I reciprocate her feelings towards me, my body returning her actions and exploring her curves. Our bodies become intertwined. I can feel myself getting turned on as her fingers brush my privates. I try to push her away, as I know that I am on my monthly and shouldn't be doing anything.

My hands and fingers explore her body over her clothes. I slowly move my hand up her stocking-clad legs, under her skirt, to her soaking wet panties. I can feel that her mound is radiating heat from excitement. Her clitoris is pulsating in reaction to my touch. I move her panties to the side and begin slipping my fingers in slowly, feeling her juices coat my fingers. While we are still connected by our lips and searching each other's bodies, she lets out quiet moans of satisfaction. My fingers and hand are still working on her mound, bringing her to the brink of orgasm and over, her muscles clenching around my fingers as the orgasm rips through her body. She manages to bring me to orgasm through my clothes – she must have guessed that I was a little reluctant to remove them.

Bo

Bo is a heterosexual woman in her thirties. She lives in rural Ireland. She has a high sex drive and usually fantasizes when she is alone. It is usually about someone she knows, often an ex. She also fantasizes about other women.

My husband is fully aware of my fantasies concerning other women, and we often used to talk about women we saw in public places, about our desires. My fantasies are usually about sex with a woman, with a man watching. The woman is not fully sure that she likes other women, but is prepared to give it a try. There are a lot of oils and touching and feeling, but saving the most important parts for last. The man is totally happy just to watch while I make this lady succumb to my ways. We play around for a long time, just kissing and fondling. The man is aroused by what he sees, but is happy to take care of his own needs while we lick each other out. The fantasy ends as a threesome.

Sharon

Sharon is a heterosexual woman in her thirties. She normally enjoys fantasizing while she is having sex with her husband. Her fantasies tend to be less about the person involved and more about the act itself. She fantasizes about people she knows, as well as strangers, men and women. She includes-teacher-and-student scenarios, threesomes and voyeurism in her list of fantasies.

I am in a brothel, with women lined up in front of me. They are standing there waiting for me to choose. They are all different shapes and all sizes: redheads, brunettes, blondes. They are all naked and they are all beautiful, but none are what I want. I call the manager over and describe what I am looking for. She takes me to a room, and I lie on the bed and wait. The wait is excruciating. I am so nervous that I feel sick – I have never been with a woman before.

When she finally arrives, she is exactly what I had

pictured in my head. Her long chocolate-brown hair is shiny, and falls in waves past her shoulders. She is not skinny like the other girls, nor is she fat. I can see through her dress, and I know that there are breasts and hips beneath it. She approaches me, and my breath catches as she kisses me on the mouth. I put my arms around her, kissing her back. My hands take on lives of their own as they explore her smooth thighs, and tremble as I open her dress.

I slowly take her clothes off her while she kisses my neck, and any part of me she can reach. I can see once she is naked that I was correct: she has a perfect hourglass figure. I put my mouth on her nipples, and I can feel them harden on my tongue. The feeling drives me wild. By now we are a tangle of limbs and the urgency is increasing. I pull away and lower myself to her crotch. She is completely hairless and licking her feels amazing. Her red manicure rakes my back as I bring her to orgasm.

And then it is my turn. She slips a finger between my legs and it feels amazing. She seems to know all the buttons to press. It only takes a moment for her to have me writhing in the bed, begging her to finish me off. She teases me, slowly slipping her finger in and out of me. I am so close and her breasts knock off my chest every time we move. It drives me crazy.

Suddenly she takes her hand away and pulls me to her. She pushes her crotch against mine. Two thrusts are all it takes, and I am there. The orgasm rushes through me and seems to last forever. When I am done, she stands, kisses me on my crotch, and flips her hair over her shoulder. Leaving her dress and underwear on the floor, she walks out.

Julie

Julie is a heterosexual woman in her thirties. She has a low sex drive. Her female friends appear a lot in her sexual fantasies, as well as threesomes and teacher-student scenarios.

I am with a friend, sitting, drinking wine, chatting and laughing. Then we start to talk about sex and what we like, laughing about how men just don't seem to understand what feels nice for us. My friend says that we would probably be better off with other women and, as we laugh, she reaches over and rubs me gently across my breast. I look at her and she looks at me, then she cups my breast and rubs it. She moves closer and opens my top, pushing my breast out of my bra and beginning to kiss, lick and suck me. I reach out and move my hand along the outside of her jeans, touching where I know it feels good.

Before I know it, we are almost naked on her couch. She is pushing her fingers against my pussy, and I am massaging both her breasts and sucking on one of her nipples. We spend a lot of time fondling, kissing, exploring. She lies down, removes her underwear, and this is it – the moment I have always waited for. She holds my head and pushes it down between her legs to her warm, delicious pussy. I can't believe that at last I am doing something I have always thought about. I lick her wet pussy, savouring the moment.

Madge

Madge is a heterosexual woman in her thirties. She lives in rural Ireland. She has a high sex drive and regularly reads erotica. She is married, and mostly fantasizes while having sex. The object of her fantasy is most often a woman who is uninhibited, sexy, vivacious and outgoing, and who will do anything and everything.

I am asleep beside the pool when a woman arrives and spots me lying on a sunbed. I am, of course, my slimmest, most fabulous self and am hard to resist, especially as I am unaware of anyone observing me. The woman is drawn to me, and comes over and kneels beside the sunlounger. She runs her fingertips up my stomach, to the valley between my breasts. My nipples harden as she pulls my bikini top open, and starts sucking on my nipples. I groan and move, getting aroused even as I sleep.

She slowly moves her mouth down over my stomach, tracing kisses as she gets lower, to my bikini bottoms. She kisses my mound through the fabric, and I wake up, extremely aroused. We kiss and my hands roam all over her upper body – breasts bared, nipples hard and rubbing against each other. Bikini bottoms are untied and dropped to the floor. She spreads my legs and kneels between them, as I tell her that I have never had a woman as a lover before.

She lowers her mouth to my labia and, with a flat tongue, licks me from top to bottom, before giving my clitoris some attention. I can feel the orgasm building inside of me even before she penetrates me with her tongue and fingers. She stops moving her tongue and teases me with the tip of her finger, gently tracing figure of eights over my clitoris and vagina.

She then moves her knees on either side of my head, so that I can taste her and get her as worked up as I am. I copy every move she made and get closer to orgasm. I am barely holding on. She is magnificent. We turn to a sixty-nine and work each other up into a frenzy. The orgasms finally explode from both of us. We lie there curled up against each other before beginning again.

Christine

Christine is a heterosexual woman in her late teens or twenties. She lives in rural Ireland. She has a very high sex drive and believes that she is a very good lover. She is in a relationship. She normally has her sexual fantasies before having sex.

I don't think I'm gay or bisexual but, then again, you might never know. In my sexual fantasies – which I always have when I'm alone – I often think about having sex with a woman. Even typing this turns me on, but I never meet women that I want to have sex with. Maybe that sounds weird, maybe it's just suppressed, I don't know, but that's how I am. I have a healthy, fairly normal sexual relationship with my boyfriend, and he doesn't know about my lesbian fantasies. He'd probably love it, but I'm afraid that if I tell him he will want me to act them out with him watching! I don't think I could do this in real life.

My lesbian fantasy always includes a very feminine, beautiful, long-haired, busty woman. She is very experienced and leads me through it. It's always very tender and slow, where my other fantasies involving men are faster and more urgent. It is never rushed. It always starts with kissing, and very slowly moves to taking our clothes off. There is no conversation at all, just touching. We don't use any sex toys or anything like that, it's all just using our hands and bodies. Even as I type this, I am becoming aroused by it. It does make me wonder about my sexual orientation, but I think it's kind of normal for women. Isn't it? The thought of our breasts and hard nipples touching, with my hand following the line of her waist and hips, really gets me going.

Sex with a Stranger

Sarah

Sarah is a heterosexual woman in her forties. She is single, and has submitted several fantasies for this book. She lives in rural Ireland and rates herself as a very good lover. She mostly fantasizes when she is alone and usually about someone she knows.

My most frequent recurring fantasy over the years has been one of me as a stripper or pole dancer. The club that I'm dancing in is full of men from my life. These men are usually ex-lovers, friends, men that wanted me but that I wasn't interested in (just to frustrate them further) and, most importantly, the ones that got away. The stage is mine, they can't get enough of my dancing, I work that pole like a pro. I finish up in front of them all, completely naked and horny as hell. Still on stage, I make myself cum, then I hand-pick one of the crowd to take to the private-dance room and fuck me.

Natalie

Natalie is a heterosexual woman in her late teens or twenties. She is single and lives in rural Ireland. She has a high sex drive and regularly reads erotica. She regularly fantasizes about a tall, dark and brooding type of man, who 'radiates masculinity'. Women don't feature in her fantasies.

My sexual fantasies are thoughts I carry with me everywhere: when I am on the bus watching passers-by, when I am in the canteen at work, or when I am doing something simple like laundry. Sometimes I get triggered by scents, like a sexy-smelling man, or when I see a hot guy pushing weights at the gym and sweating. Sometimes the closeness of a stranger on a bus, especially a man, can set me off. I imagine frantic, lustful sex, sex that is a consummation of everything: my body, breath and soul. I like the element of surprise, like a boyfriend coming up from behind, and blowing on and kissing my neck while he pulls roughly at my nipples. It gets me wet anticipating being on all fours, taking in all of him, feeling him stretch me and fuck me until I lose everything, him knowing that I can go further, and making me do exactly that.

My second favourite is stranger sex, like meeting a hot stranger at a work function and making the sort of eye contact that says it all. We carry on with the boring chit-chat, discussing formalities, while I know that he knows what I know: that sex is inevitable. I love thinking about the delay of sex. The flirtation takes on a painful quality, as I wait for him to finally submit to his wanting, hard dick – to stop everything and just take me. The elevator ride is exquisite: the mouth-on-mouth consumption, the hands-on approach, the feel of his hard cock pushing against my vagina. I like to think about us on a table, how the need in us is so bad that he rips off my tights and hoists up my skirt while I quickly take off my top. I undo the buttons of his shirt while we're kissing, laughing as he tries to wriggle out of his jacket, freeing his strong arms. I am happy knowing what is coming.

I take his belt off slowly, enjoying teasing him, hearing his excited breath when he feels me through my knickers, all wet just for him. I take his dick quickly in my hands and then I go down his slide, slowing down only when I know that I am going to explode, to keep the tension hot. I bite him softly as my moaning takes over. Afterwards, I always end up totally spent.

Kathleen

Kathleen is a bisexual woman in her late teens or twenties. She has a high sex drive and considers herself to be a very good lover. She is currently single, and has a variety of fantasies, including private dancing, voyeurism and threesomes with two women. Her fantasies change all the time. She gets bored with

*them as they're only fantasies, and so completely new, more
interesting fantasies regularly pop into her head.*

Táim ag ócáid lán le daoine saibhre nach bhfuil aithne agam
orthu; chuaigh mé mar ghar do chara, agus tá sise sáite i
gcómhra le grúpa sa seomra eile. Tá cineál leadrán orm ach
táim sásta ag súil timpeall ag breathnú ar an
seanfhoirgneamh álainn atá san óstán seo.

Ansin feicim spéirbhean ina seasamh in aice na tine.
Bean cosúil le Nigella Lawson le breathnú atá inti agus tá
éad orm ar chibé fear atá chun an gúna sin atá uirthi a
bhaint ag deireadh na hoíche agus a corp nocht a fheiceáil
ina iomláine.

Tá sí ina aonar cosúil liom féin agus beartaím labhairt léi
cé nach gceapann go bhfaighidh mé mórán as. Tarlaíonn
sé, áfach, go bhfuil go réitímid go maith agus ní rófhada go
dtí go bhfuil an beirt againn ag gáire le chéile.

Ansin tosaím ag insint di faoin foirgneamh, cé chomh
sean is atá sé agus is ar nós go bhfuil suim aici. Deir sí go
bhfuil sí ag fanacht sa suite agus ar mhaith liom é a fheiceáil? D'fhán JFK sa suite sin cheana agus mar sin chuaigh
mé suas chun feiceáil.

Nílimid sa seomra ach cúpla soicind nuair a chuireann
sí mé suite ar an leaba agus gan aon rud a rá osclaíonn sí cúl
a gúna agus titeann sé ar an urlár. Fobhrístí lása atá ar a corp
griandaite. Mothaím drithlín idir mo dhá chos agus cuimh-
ním nach bhfuil aon fobhrístí orm faoi mo ghúna ar chor ar
bith. Insíonn sí dom go bhfuil orm an gúna a bhaint agus
tríocha soicind i ndiaidh sin taim nocht ar a leaba ag

breathnú uirthi ag breathnú orm, an bheirt againn ag anáil go trom sa chiúnas.

Cuireann sí a lámh ar a chíochbheart féin, ag tarraingt fáine timpeall a dide. Seasaim, le drúis, ach stopaim, gan a bheith cinnte céard is ceart dom a dhéanamh léi fiú. Cuireann sí a lámh ar mo bhásta agus bogaim níos gaire di, mo teanga ag rith timpeall mo bhéal le drúis. Tá a beola mín ar mo bheola agus bogann sí a teanga go mall timpeall mo bhéil. Tá mo chorp ag bogadh go nádúrtha ina treo, tonn i ndiaidh toinne.

Táim cinnte go bhfuil mé fliuch báite. Tá sí go maith, tuigeann sí nach bhfuilim cinnte céard le déanamh agus tugann sí treoracha. Baineann a cíochbheart ar dtús agus cuirim mo bhéal timpeall a didi. Ligeann sí torann beag teacht amach as a bhéal agus tosaíonn sí ag anáil níos tapúla. Mothaím mo bhrillín ag preabadh; teastaíonn sí uaim. Ag pógadh a boilg, téim ar mo ghlúine agus bainim a fobhrístí di, thíos a chosa míne. Tá an boladh ag teacht uaithi go hálainn.

Go mall cuirim méar óna himleacán go dtí a bhrillí, síos go dtí go mothaím an leacht. Craitheann sí ach ní dhéanaim níos mó. Seasaim arís agus insíonn sí dom gur léir go bhfuil a treoir ag teastáil uaim agus go mbeidh sise i gceannais ar an oíche seo. Is deacair mo aird a choimead ar aon áit amháin agus ise ag siúil go dtí an cófra. Feicim a tóin don chéad uair díreach sula chasann sí, fuip ina lámh aici.

Sharon

Sharon is a heterosexual woman in her thirties. She normally enjoys fantasizing while she is having sex. Her fantasies tend to be less about the person involved, and more about the act itself. She is married, and has submitted several fantasies to this book.

I am lying on my bed, naked and with my legs wide apart. The stranger stands above me. He is tall, handsome and looks incredibly strong. He is wearing black trousers and a crisp white shirt. I can see his erection forming as he looks at me. I smile at him, and he takes that as an invitation to unbutton his shirt. I am already aroused. There is a tingling between my legs, and I can feel myself getting wet. My hips have a life of their own, moving without my permission. I am squirming with desire. He takes off his shirt.

I reach up and open his trousers, freeing his erection. He climbs onto the bed and, on all fours, takes a hard nipple into his mouth. I gasp with pleasure, and he lowers himself onto me. I reach around and put my hands on his tight bum. I squeeze, and pull him to me. I can feel his erection against my wet pussy. He teases me with his dick, spreading my wetness up and down. I am gasping with desire. I try to pull him into me but he pulls back, teasing me until I cannot take it anymore. When he finally enters me it is sudden, and feels amazing. His first few thrusts are urgent, and I am getting closer and closer. Just as I am about to cum, he slows.

I feel incredibly frustrated and pull him deeper into me. His thrusts are now slow and deliberate. It feels amazing. I can feel that he is close too. We are slippery with perspiration, and our chests slide easily against each other. I start to cum and it is slow, prolonged and excruciating. He feels me tighten around him, and this spurs him to orgasm too. He calls my name over and over as he does.

Karen

Karen is a heterosexual woman in her forties. She normally fantasizes when she is alone, usually about strangers, never about women. She is married, and her fantasies include exhibitionism, force fantasies, voyeurism and domination.

My husband and I were very adventurous in the earlier part of our relationship. There isn't a part of the house that we haven't done it in. We generally still have a healthy sex life, albeit not as exciting – it's more predictable. I think what turns me on about my fantasy is the element of surprise.

I'm asleep when an intruder comes into my bedroom. He blindfolds me and ties my hands to the bedpost. I struggle with him but then he starts to fondle my breasts. When he sees me becoming aroused, he starts licking and sucking them. He moves down my body and between my legs before getting on top of me, and then fucks me hard and fast until I have my first orgasm. He unties me and turns me over, and again fucks me hard and fast. All the while, he is saying, 'Give it to me you dirty whore', as I am groaning. He finally grabs my hair and pulls me back onto him, pinching my nipples, and my whole body goes into the most amazing orgasm. He throws me back down on the bed, still blindfolded, and leaves. Then my husband comes in and asks what happened, and I just can't tell him.

Isabella

Isabella is a heterosexual woman in her thirties. She lives in rural Ireland. She doesn't rate herself very highly as a lover. She usually fantasizes when she is alone, but also while she is having sex. She usually thinks about a stranger when she is fantasizing. He is confident and successful in all aspects of his life. He is charming but forceful, and pursues her.

I feel very boring and not very experienced. When I think about sex with the sexual partners I have had so far, I feel it was 'wham, bam'. I never thought sex could be more than that. I would quite happily never have it again if it was always going to be like that.

I have often thought about catching the eye of a stranger while travelling. In my fantasy, he is older than me, and certainly more experienced. We get chatting and the chemistry is explosive. I decide to go for it and ask him for a drink. After the drink, he takes me to his room. He stands behind me and moves my hair, slowly blowing on my neck, and then kisses my back and unzips my dress. He undresses me slowly, lays me on the bed and kisses me from my feet to my underwear. I can tell that he is very aroused. He slowly pulls off my panties and gently enters me, moving in ways I could only imagine. I feel my body succumb to the movements and experiences that I have never felt before. I bite my lip as we move in unison, then scream out in exhilaration. He keeps kissing me all over my body.

After we sleep for a while, he takes me by the hand and

leads me to the shower. We lather each other up and both become stimulated. Then he picks me up, takes me to the bed and we have sex again. In the morning, I go before he wakes, leaving him a note. Time for me to get back to reality.

Linda

Linda is a heterosexual woman in her late teens or twenties. She is in a relationship with the only man she has ever slept with. She has a very high sex drive and usually fantasizes while she is alone, about a stranger. He is a tall man with long, black hair tied at the base of his neck. He's muscular and wears all black, with black boots.

I've only had sex with one person, my current boyfriend. Before I had sex, I never thought about what would come after, or ways of spicing it up, but that's how it is now. When I daydream about sex, it's not my boyfriend that I'm thinking of but a stranger: a tall handsome stranger with desire in his eyes only for me. I read erotica, so my fantasy is probably influenced by that.

I'm lying in bed in a hotel room. I feel like someone has been watching me, but when I look around I can't see anything. I'm guessing it is just jitters from being in a different place on my own. I'm lying in bed and can't help but get aroused. I order some porn for myself; I need to pleasure myself, I need to feel what the porn stars are 'feeling'. I pull down my trousers and open my shirt a bit, and I start rubbing. I'm going faster and faster and I'm just about to—I stop.

Suddenly I feel those eyes on me again.

I look at the doorway, and there he is: a tall man, with long black hair tied at the base of his neck, his strong-looking arms catching the light. He has just the right amount of muscle. He's wearing a tight black T-shirt, dark black jeans and black boots. I can feel the heat of his stare on me. My hand is frozen, my breathing suddenly low and raspy, as I look at this mysterious man. Neither of us says a word, but I'm drawn to him, a deep ache in me needs him. I have to have him. He takes a step forward and the light catches his face, his eyes. I can't look away. He has such heat and desire in his eyes that he makes me instantly wet. He looks at my hand and says, 'Oh baby no, let me take care of you.'

He moves forward, slow but determined, his eyes trailing over my body. He bites his lip, and I groan. He moves on top of me and captures my mouth, moving my hand, taking over. We last all night, doing everything there is to do, in every possible position. He's rough but tender, showing me that he's the man, that he is strong. He makes me tremble with excitement and I can't get enough of him. All night long he shows me what a real man can do; he shows me how naughty I really am.

Deirdre

Deirdre is a bisexual woman in her late teens or twenties. She is single and, despite a low sex drive, rates herself as a good lover. She regularly reads erotica and enjoys her sexual fantasies when she is alone. She usually fantasizes about sex with a stranger, but also about being watched, threesomes with men (and with women) and domination.

I am alone in an office. A man comes in. He walks up to me, kisses me passionately and throws me onto the desk. He takes off my underwear and works his lips from between my legs to my neck while he undresses me. He fucks me softly, then harder, and when he is done he leaves me his business card.

One-Night Stand

Jeanne

Jeanne is a heterosexual woman in her thirties. She usually fantasizes when she is alone, and always about a one-night stand with someone she vaguely knows. Her fantasies never include her boyfriend. There are a few men (and women) who come up regularly in her fantasies.

This fantasy is one I have regularly. I switch the man in it, depending on my mood. Lately I've been fantasizing about a neighbour who is looking particularly hot at the moment. Whatever it is, it's working; he is gorgeous. I know him to say hi to, but we wouldn't be friends.

In my fantasy, it's a Friday evening in the summer. We have all gone to the pub after work. Everyone's in great form, and there's that lovely feeling of the weekend stretched out ahead of us. My neighbour is in his usual spot at the bar, chatting to his friends. He works on a farm and spends a lot of time outdoors, so he has a lovely tan. He is wearing a white shirt and blue jeans. The shirt is slightly open at the top, and I can see his chest hair peeking out. He is so manly – broad-shouldered and strong. I can't stop looking over at him, and he keeps catching my eye. I look away shyly every time he does, but my heart is racing.

I walk past him to go to the ladies, and he says hello as I brush by. On my way back, he is looking out for me and, as I pass, he puts his hand on my ass and says hello. The pub is packed so noone can see where his hand is. I am shocked and thrilled at the same time. I'm not interested in starting a relationship with this guy, so I'm not playing the long game – I just want a night of fun.

As I stand there talking to him we both know that at some point in the night I am going to have my way with him, and he with me. The night continues, with us flirting and chatting every time we end up near each other. I can't keep my mind on any of the conversations with my friends as I am so caught up in thinking about how we are going to have sex very soon.

As the night comes to an end, I drop my spare key into his pocket. I whisper the number of my apartment in his ear, and tell him that I'll be waiting for him. I leave with my friends and head home as normal – none of them have any idea what I'm up to. I get home and change into a sexy silk nightie, with suspenders and knickers. I light a few candles.

I am so turned on by this stage that I can't wait to hear that key in the door.

I am not disappointed; the key turns in the door and then he is standing there, with a bulging erection and a cheeky smile.

'Well, well,' he says as he shuts the door. 'Aren't you a sight for sore eyes.'

I walk over, totally in control, and slowly take off his jacket, letting it fall to the floor. He stays totally still as I allow my lips to brush over his, teasing him. Then he takes me, and we kiss passionately as I rip off his clothes. His body is as muscular and toned as I had suspected. He lifts me to the couch, and kisses me all over. He leaves my nightie on, unclips my suspenders, pushes my knickers to the side and starts teasing me with his tongue. Then he takes my knickers off completely, pulling them down with his teeth. I am really wet; I need to feel him inside me.

I take off his boxers and admire his beautiful, wide penis – one of the biggest I've ever seen. I make him lie on his back as I go down on him. He groans with pleasure as I take him in my mouth. Before I go too far and lose him to an orgasm, I sit up and straddle him, allowing the head of his penis to rub against my clit. He massages my breasts and begs me to take him in. I hold his gaze and slowly allow him to enter me. We are both moaning at this stage, both close to orgasm. I take it slowly to make it last. The feeling of his penis as it makes its way deeper and deeper inside of me is driving me crazy. He is fully inside me now, and we are screaming with pleasure. My orgasm is long and intense and beautiful.

He flips me over and really goes for it, pounding me with every ounce of energy he has. Watching him over me – broad and muscular and all man – makes me horny even as my orgasm subsides. I can feel the familiar build-up and, as he explodes inside of me, I cum again. Our bodies are wet with sweat as we lie there, exhausted.

We both know that this won't happen again; the thrill of winning each other will not be there after this. We make the most of it and spend the night shagging until day breaks. We have a shower and say goodbye, our lips sore from kissing, our bodies exhausted from sex. No one will ever know except us what an amazing night we had.

Lola

Lola is a heterosexual woman in her thirties. She has a very high sex drive and mostly fantasizes when she is alone. She sometimes fantasizes about people she knows, or ex-lovers. She fantasizes about sexual encounters in her past, like this one.

So I end up going out on a hot summer's night – totally unplanned. I was eating ice cream on the beach at 10:30 PM when I got a call to meet some friends. I really wasn't in the mood to go, but remembered that it was a friend's birthday and felt obliged to attend. Besides, I knew a certain someone who would be there, and who I shouldn't want to see but still did. I came home, had a quick shower and spontaneously decided to shave my legs and trim my bikini line. I put on a pair of soft maroon shorts and a pink T-shirt with sandals. I got to the bar, and in walks that guy I was supposed to not like; someone that on paper did not 'tick the boxes'. I would find out later that he ticked them all.

We said a polite hello. I had met him before. I think he had half-tried to make a move on me once, but had never plucked up the courage. He asked if we wanted to check out the music inside. There was something about this guy – I still can't put my finger on it to this day, but the chemistry between us was electrifying. When I think about him, I call him 'Time-Warp Boy'. He asked me a simple question that I can't remember, but his eyes said, 'I want to fuck you.' It didn't matter what was verbal, the body language was overpowering. I felt like everyone in the room must have known we were going to fuck that night.

We moved into the gig room. We had never spoken much before that night, but he made an effort to talk. We could tell by looking into each other's eyes that it was only a matter of time. He took me by the hand and twirled me across the dance floor; we didn't care who was looking at us. When everyone stopped moving, he moved closer and tugged at the bottom of my shorts, near my bum.

Time-Warp Boy moved around the floor for a little bit but kept coming back over to me, mostly just making eye contact. It didn't take long, but it felt like an eternity. He came over again, looked me straight in the eye and said, 'I want to make you cum.' I felt my knees go weak and my pussy become instantly wet. I was in shock. Nobody had ever been so brazen, and I loved it.

Everyone planned to go to a friend's house for the birthday

party. Time-Warp Boy and I said we would pick up some drinks in mine and meet them later. We never made it. When we arrived back at mine, we smoked and drank under the stars, and then he told me to sit on his lap. I did. He started stroking me, sliding his hands under my shorts, near my underwear. I told him we needed to be careful in case the neighbours were watching but he kept going.

We kissed for a while, and then it was time to go inside – we both knew what was coming. The excitement was phenomenal and the anticipation was exquisite. We went into my room, took off each other's clothes, and more or less crash-landed on the bed. The energy and intensity we each had for one other was positively animalistic, raw. It felt like this was exactly how sex was supposed to be. Time-Warp Boy knew what he was doing, all the way. Sucking, pulling, kissing, biting and caressing, changing from slow and sensual to hard, fast, intense and electrifying.

My senses were on overload in the best way possible. He started rolling my nipples between his finger and thumb and offered me his cock to suck. At the same time he was pushing his fingers inside me. His dick was rock-solid, long and beautiful. I loved it. He then lifted my legs high over my head and pushed his cock inside me – slowly at first, then, once inside, he began pummelling me so hard the headboard started banging loudly. He then pulled back, lifted my hips up at an angle for deeper penetration and pumped me hard. His long hair got in the way a few times. I pushed it back as I wanted to see his face.

We moved positions again, and I got on top of him. Normally I don't feel as confident in this position, but he had awoken all my senses and I felt like a goddess with him, so all my inhibitions just disappeared. I guided his cock inside me and started to move slowly. I started to circulate my hips around, then moved them and up and down, faster and faster, which made him groan with pleasure. He grabbed both of my breasts and rubbed my nipples, leaning forward to suck them. He threw me aside again and pulled me in front of him so that he was behind me. In one swift move, he used one of his knees to push my legs apart. He moved closer to me, pushed my back down so my ass was up high and my head was resting on the bed, and pushed his dick inside me. Soon we were in sync, and as he started pushing into me harder and harder, he started spanking my ass, and then pinching and pumping me at the same time. He put his finger up my ass – it felt amazing.

He leaned forwards and pulled me back by my hair. Then we looked into each other's eyes and had a slow French kiss. He had one hand on my breast and one hand on my throat and his dick inside me. He pushed my head down again, pulled my ass back onto his cock and fucked me hard. I think my eyeballs rolled into the back of my head I came so hard. What a night.

Anastasia

Anastasia is a heterosexual woman in her late teens or twenties. She is single and hasn't yet had a serious relationship. She has a high sex drive and a crush on a man, who she fantasizes about. She is still a virgin but loves to masturbate. She would

like to lose her virginity with someone she knows, who she is
comfortable with.

I'm out at a bar. I'm wearing a sexy dress with no bra, just a
G-string and heels. I look sexy and feel sexy. You can see my
nipples through my dress. It's busy and I am aware that
everyone is looking at me. The man I have a crush on is at
the bar with his friends. He sees me walk in. We make eye
contact and I can feel my pulse racing. It's coming towards
the end of the night and we've both been drinking. He
approaches me and we start talking. It's normal chit-chat,
but we both flirt. He's standing close to me now, and the bar
is busy. He puts his hand on my lower back and then onto
my ass. I feel wet. We decide to get a taxi and leave.

Not much happens in the taxi,. We kiss and he puts his
hand on my inner thigh. We arrive at his place. As soon as
we get inside, I reach for him and we start kissing again. It's
really heated, we are both aroused and want to have sex there
and then. I brush him off and we go into the kitchen. I hop
up on the counter and he comes over to me. We flirt and
laugh, we both want this to happen. I have my legs wrapped
around him and we start kissing again. I can feel that he is
hard. I whisper to him that we should go to the bedroom. He
leads me to his room and closes the door. I walk around,
looking at his things. I look up and we stare at each other. I
lift my hand, signalling him to come over to me.

When he holds me, I lay myself down on the bed with
him on top of me. He is between my legs, so I start thrusting
against him, making him know I want him. I pull off his shirt

and start undoing his belt. I kiss him on his neck and chest. He slides the straps off my shoulders and my dress falls off. I lay back and he pulls it off over my feet. I keep my heels on; I like it that way. He kisses me on the lips, then my breasts and my inner thighs. He rips off my G-string and puts it in his back pocket. He starts going down on me. It is unreal.

I moan; I have never felt pleasure like this before. He grabs my breast while he's still going down on me. He looks up and lifts me: I'm now on top of him. I pull down his jeans and grab his penis. It's long and hard, which makes me so horny. I put it inside myself and start moving my body. He has his hands on my hips, guiding me. We are looking into each other's eyes, the pleasure is coming.

We both explode. I'm moaning. He makes a grunt which turns me on more. I stay in that position and he puts his hand on my neck. I fall beside him and we kiss passionately. We sleep, with him holding me.

Stephanie

Stephanie is a heterosexual woman in her late teens or twenties. She lives in rural Ireland and has a very high sex drive. She thinks about sex everywhere, including when she's at work. She has a recurring fantasy about a man she knows. He is tall, and dark-haired with green-blue eyes and a sporty build. He dresses well. He has a great job and travels overseas a lot with work. He is seven years older than her, and smokes – she loves a man who smokes.

I know Mr J is based in the city due to work, and I happen to be staying for a week. I let him know of my whereabouts. He suggests we meet. I agree, and he books one of the well-known hotels. He names a time and a room. I make sure I am well dressed for the occasion, thinking along the lines of Beyoncé's 'Partition' video: stockings, suspenders, thong, bra, heels and coat. I make my way to the hotel feeling nervous. I've always wanted to dress up for a man – especially in a hotel room, especially for him.

I let myself in and there he is, sitting on the edge of the bed, just in his shirt and trousers. I walk towards him,. God he looks good and he smells great. He slowly runs his hands up my stockings, then his thumb along my thong. I start to get wet and I just want to jump on him. He removes my coat and lets it fall to the ground. What is he going to do with me? This is the first time we have met, he is older and this is intimidating me. He kisses me – hot and heavy with plenty of tongue – then makes his way down my neck and onto my breasts. It feels amazing. He removes my bra while kissing me, teasing me with his tongue.

I remove his shirt, skin-on-skin, my nipples rubbing against his chest. He places me on the bed and removes his trousers. I am really wet now and just want him inside me. He takes an ice cube, rubs it round my lips and down my neck, over my torso, teasing me. I kiss him from his neck down to his chest, around his navel and then back up and down again, teasing him. I pull down his boxers to reveal his erection. I gently place my hot, moist mouth on it, slowly sucking and moving my tongue around it so that he can't take anymore.

He scoops me up and lifts me against the wall, where he removes my suspenders and thong. He places himself inside me; he is big and throbbing. We are both sweating now, this feels so dirty and I am letting him fill me. I can't believe this is happening, but it is well worth the wait.

Molly

Molly is a heterosexual woman in her late teens or twenties. She has a high sex drive. She sometimes fantasizes about other women, but also about attractive men she knows.

I love the thought of meeting a stranger through online dating and being really aroused and turned on by him. I've never tried online dating, and I often fantasize about strangers. In my fantasy, I meet a guy for a drink and it is obvious from the start that we are into each other. We get a taxi back to his place. There is no talking. He leads me to his front room, where he immediately grabs me, bends me over and pulls up my dress. He doesn't kiss me. He rubs himself against me, getting very erect. He undresses me completely, ordering me to get up on the table and play with myself for him. He takes a chair and sits down in front of me, very close so that he can get a good view, all the while playing with himself and talking dirty to me. I continue to play with myself until he can't take not touching me anymore, and he uses his tongue to bring me to orgasm.

Superior Sex:
Boss, Trainer, Teacher

Ruby

Ruby is a lesbian in her late teens or twenties. She is in a relationship. She has a very high sex drive and fantasizes mostly when she is alone. The person she fantasizes most often about is a yoga instructor. Men sometimes feature in her fantasies, as do threesomes with other women, sex with strangers and domination.

I've had this fantasy for a few years now, and I often think about it when I'm alone. It was only when I saw it played out in pornography that my imagination really ran wild with it.

I walk into a gym, into one of those private side studio rooms surrounded with mirrors, and I see a naked woman lying flat on the floor. She's always curvy and sexy, but also heathy and toned. She slowly brings her leg towards her chest and holds it there for several seconds before releasing it slowly. The fantasy continues with this woman in front of me practicing all the typical yoga positions (downward dog really gets me), only she's completely naked. I never once make contact with her, I am only an observer.

The peak for me is when I fantasize about her taking out one of those exercise balls. She lies across it on her stomach and rolls back and forth. She never treats the situation as erotic, no sexy faces, no winking, no nothing. It is literally this woman doing yoga naked. Such a soothing and relaxing practice combined with something so erotic really pushes my buttons.

Lizzie

Lizzie is a heterosexual woman in her late teens or twenties. She is in a relationship and regularly reads erotica. Her sexual fantasies happen when she is alone, as well as before and during sex.

It's a school scenario. I am being punished for something I've done wrong, in front of the whole school. The teacher orders me to lean over the gym horse and raise my skirt. With a flesh-jiggling *whap*, she brings the paddle down onto my bottom. Again and again, she brings the paddle down onto my buttocks, with the whole school watching behind me. Then she orders me to remove my knickers.

Burning with humiliation, I drop them to the floor and step out of them.

'Turn back to the horse,' she orders.

I acquiesce, my naked bottom and pussy exposed to the school. More wince-inducing spanks land on my rear, and I cry out in pain, while simultaneously feeling my juices drip down my legs. The teacher steps back, a malicious sneer twisting across her face.

'Look at that,' she snarls, 'she's enjoying it. Get up.'

Trembling, I pull myself to my feet. I reach for my discarded panties on the floor, but she snatches them away before I can get there, folding them neatly into her pocket, eyes travelling along my wet, quivering thighs.

'Back to class,' she barks. 'All of you.'

I open my mouth to ask if I may return to the dorm for a fresh pair of underwear, but, as if she has read my mind, the teacher sneers, 'You too madam. Now.' Cheeks flaming with humiliation, I trail my classmates back to class. Our uniform skirts come almost to the knee, but I burn with embarrassed, self-consciousness as I try to maintain what is left of my dignity as we return to class.

In class, I keep my head down, but I hear the other girls sniggering, and see the boys leering as I traipse past. My bottom sears with pain in the hard chairs, but I bite back the tears and longingly look forward to the end of day when I can return to the dorm and lie face down in the dark, alone. When the bell signals the end of day the others stream into the dining room, common rooms or sport pitches, but I rush straight to the dorms. The sheets of my bed are a cool relief. I bury my face into my pillow and sigh as the cool air soothes my flesh.

'Well, well, well.'

The voice makes me freeze. It is a deep, authoritative voice, and I know it.

'Now young lady, you know you are not allowed to be up here at this time.'

Hastily, I reach to pull down my skirt. A hand on my bottom stops me, large and firm and mercifully cool.

'What's this?' the man's voice asks. 'Miss Marcy's special punishment?'

I nod and turn my head, meeting the eye of the gym teacher behind me.

'Well now, I'm sure you wouldn't want more of this, would you?'

He holds eye contact as he talks, his hand squeezing and sliding over my bottom. I shake my head.

'Which you know would be meted out if you were found to be here . . . '

His fingers slip between my legs, sliding along my slit, finding a slick wetness there.

'Please don't tell,' I whisper. 'I'll do anything.'

'Anything, eh?' His voice is curious.

'Anything . . . '

I hear the zip of his trousers come down. I turn, already mentally preparing myself for his cock in my mouth, but his hand on my back pushes me firmly back to the bed.

'No, no,' he says, 'we can't have you turning around, risking further injury.'

His fingers slip further up my leg, finding my clitoris. I gasp then groan as he rubs it steadily, expertly with his finger. I have dreamt of the gym teacher, with his blond hair and soaring cheekbones, so many times that I cannot believe this is really happening. I hold my breath as his thick, strong fingers slide inside me. Two of them fill me up, and he stimulates my G spot until I feel like I'm going to cum, and I think how weird it would be to orgasm on a teacher's hand.

Suddenly he withdraws his fingers, and I cry out in protest. But he is not finished. Instead he draws me to my knees, spreading them out so that my whole pussy is exposed to him. He dives in face first, and I groan as his tongue slides up and down my slit, slipping inside me, tickling my clit, his lips wrapping around it, sucking on it and driving me wild. Then he is on the bed behind me, my knickers are around my knees, and I hold my breath as he presses the head of his cock against my slit and pushes in. It is tight, but he has made me so wet that, with a couple of pushes, his whole dick slides inside of me, filling me up. He begins to fuck me wildly from behind, hitting spots I never knew existed.

The pleasure is extraordinary, like nothing I have ever felt before, and as he reaches around to grab my tits, kneading my breasts through my shirt while he hammers into me from behind, I feel myself coming over and over again, and I cry out with pleasure, clinging to the headboard for dear life, wishing he would never stop. But as my pussy clamps and contracts around him, he cries out and buries himself deep inside me. I feel hot jets of his cum stream into me.

I don't move, trying to catch my breath. Slowly, he withdraws, leaving me devastatingly empty and yet wonderfully full, as our cum trails down the inside of my thigh. He strokes my bottom gently, but the pain has all gone by now.

'I won't tell,' he whispers, 'I promise.'

Claire

Claire is a heterosexual woman in her thirties. She has a high sex drive and lives in rural Ireland. From time to time she reads erotica and currently fantasizes a lot about her boss. This fantasy is about him.

The phone rings. I glance quickly across my desk to see the extension number. It's him.

'Can you call down to go through those figures?' he asks.

I walk down the hall to his office, both nervous and excited. I'm wearing a short grey skirt, a fitted black shirt, lace top hold-ups and black high heels. As I open the door and walk into his office, I see his eyes move up from the screen to me. We greet each other politely and he gives me one of his warm smiles. I sit down and he gets up from his desk to walk to the other side of the large meeting table. He looks good, very good.

My mouth is already dry as we begin to talk about the work at hand, but I can't help but get side-tracked. I get side-tracked by his smile, sometimes sweet, sometimes cheeky, and by his hair. It's dark, but with some grey. It suits him, and I like it. At one point, he hands me some paper and his hand brushes against mine. I can't help but wonder what his hand would feel like touching my body in places bosses aren't supposed to touch.

Taking off his designer glasses and placing them on the table, he sits back in the chair with his hands behind his head. *How am I supposed to discuss work when he looks this good?* I think to myself. Eventually, when the work is complete, I pick up my notepad and pen to leave and push my chair neatly back under the table.

As I turn around to walk towards the door, I notice out of the corner of my eye that instead of going back to his desk, he turns in my direction and follows me. I pretend not to notice and continue towards the door. Just as I touch the handle, I feel his hand touch my arm, and I hear him say my name. I turn around, expecting him to give me some more paperwork. Instead, for what feels like minutes but is really just seconds, he pauses and looks at me. Eventually, he speaks.

'Is it just me, or do you feel like there is something between us?'

My knees feel weak, but I somehow manage to stay vertical. I try to sound casual.

'What do you mean?'

Inside, I know exactly what he means.

'I think you know what I mean,' he says, and takes a step closer to me as I reluctantly step back in the opposite direction towards the door. I want to rip his shirt off right there and then but I know I shouldn't and I somehow manage to contain my urge. I feel the door at my back. I can't go any further. He continues to move closer, until he's so close I can feel his breath.

'I can't stop thinking about you,' he says slowly. 'You're driving me crazy. It's not just me, is it?'

I think of all the things I should say, all denying it.

Instead, the words, 'No, I feel the same way', come out of my mouth. I realise what I've said and quickly say, 'But it's not right'.

'Why?' he retaliates.

'You know why,' I say to him, as firmly as I can.

He looks me in the eye, and I wait for him to say something, but instead he brings his hand up to the side of my face and carefully brushes my hair behind my ear. Then he tilts his head to the side, moves in closer and softly kisses my neck. He brushes his lips along my neck until he reaches my ear, and he says, 'This isn't right?'

I'm in heaven, it feels perfect, but, blatantly lying, I tell him, 'No, it's not right.'

With that, he tilts his head to the other side, and moves in closer to plant a perfectly soft and spine-tingling kiss on the other side of my neck. He then drifts up towards my ear again and whispers, 'And this isn't right?'

'No' I lie.

Again. He looks at me with one of his cheeky smiles, and takes the notebook from my hand, the notebook that I am holding ever so tightly. If I weren't holding onto it, there's no telling what I would have grabbed. He places it on a shelf beside us.

Knowing that I'm caving in, he looks down at my shirt

and opens the top button. He skims its edge, and moves towards the second and third buttons, opening each one. As he does, his hand brushes my skin, and I melt. He then moves my shirt and bra to one side, exposing my breast. He caresses it with his experienced touch. He knows exactly what to do. I'm enjoying it so much that I can't even try to stop him. I'm wet and he hasn't even touched me there yet. He looks me at me again and says, 'And even this isn't right?'

I can't lie anymore . . . I'm his.

'Fuck me', I beg, as he comes in for the kill, and we kiss hard and fast.

He's an amazing kisser. *Christ, isn't there anything this man can't do?* I catch him off-guard and push him so that he's up against the door.

'You're not the boss now', I inform him.

He smiles with surprise. With that I move my hand along his chest. I stop at his top button and open it. I don't want to waste any more time, I want his shirt off now. I get as far as the third button, then rip the rest of his shirt open, the rest of the buttons flying to the floor. Neither of us care. I lightly glide over his naked chest and slowly move south. I brush along the outside of his trousers, feeling the hardness of his erection beneath.

I look at him, and ask him to give me his hand. I bring it along the inside of my thigh, under my skirt and continue upwards. I push my thong to the side and I place his hand, exactly where I've wanted it for so long. He pauses for a second. I move my hand away and he begins to touch me. He strokes his thumb along my clit, with just the right amount of pressure and movement. It feels so good. Then he slides his fingers in, first one, then a second. My body tingles all over.

I groan as I bring my hand to his belt to undo it, and within seconds his clothes fall to the floor. Teasing, I lightly brush my nails along the inside of his thigh, all the way up to his manhood and barely skim along the length of his erection with my fingers. I take him by surprise when I grip him hard and start to move up and down again and again. I want him in my mouth but suddenly, he grabs my waist.

'What did you say about being the boss?' he asks.

Before I can reply, he kisses me hard while forcefully pushing me back towards the table, shoving a chair out of the way and lifting me onto the table. He quickly removes my shirt, skirt and thong, while touching me all over and sucking my nipples – sending me even closer. It's like the past few months of holding back are all coming to this one moment: we want each other and it can't happen quickly enough.

'I want to be inside you,' he sighs.

It is music to my ears – I don't think I can wait any longer. He lingers for a second, then he oh-so-slowly enters me. He fills me, and I lie back on the table in ecstasy. He begins to thrust as my body writhes in pure pleasure. I move my hand down so he's in between my fingers as I lightly caress my clit at the same time. We're close.

Eventually his rhythmic thrusting sends me into pieces. I pull him closer and scratch my nails down his back in satisfaction. He collapses into my chest as he comes inside me, calling out my name. We lay there, both trying to get our breath back. I already want to do it again . . .

Caitriona

Caitriona is a heterosexual woman in her late teens or twenties. She is single and describes herself as a good lover. She often fantasizes about a lecturer from her old college with whom she always had great chemistry – and for whom she had a good deal of respect for, academically. He was a stereotypical lecturer, with corduroy, tweeds, an English accent and a sprinkling of grey in his hair. This fantasy is about him.

I find myself in an art gallery in the dead of night and know I shouldn't be there. I can't help exploring the building, and become aware that I'm wearing a sheer, skin-tight black leotard. In the silence, I hear footsteps behind me and a throat is cleared. It's the gallery director, an older man who once lectured me in college, and with whom I had incredible chemistry. Without a word, he looks deep into my eyes and picks me up, carrying me to his office. I try to fight him off, but I know that it's pointless, he's too strong.

He fucks everything off his desk and throws me onto it. I see his crisp shirt, feel his eyes all over me and smell the scent that had driven me wild years ago. I also feel his hard-on rubbing up against me, driving me mad. The leotard is unceremoniously ripped from my body. He holds me down, pinning me to the desk. I can feel my wetness dripping down my thighs. His lips explore my body, and he tells me not to move, but I can't resist the urge to move my body rhythmically with his as he teases my nipples with his lips and tongue.

As punishment for moving he bites down on my inner thigh, hard. I fight between the natural movement of my body and the pain of his biting, and the more he bites the more wild I'm driven. I feel exhilarated and break free, pinning him down on the desk, sitting on his face and telling him to shut the fuck up. I'm dizzy from his teasing, but empowered by feeling on top and in control. Our face-fucking leads to his glorious cock taking me on his huge, shiny oak desk, just like the one we used to flirt across years before.

Ellie

Ellie is a heterosexual woman in her late teens or twenties. She is single and describes her sex drive as average. She normally fantasizes about someone she knows. At the moment she fantasizes regularly about her muscly, strong-armed trainer at the gym.

I'm doing a boxing training session in a private room in the gym with my trainer. There's been a lot of flirting and some serious sexual tension between us, and it's getting intense. Sweat is dripping off my face and rolling down my back. I get really into it, and when I look up at him, he just grabs me and kisses me passionately. I wrap my arms around his neck and he shoves me against the wall, pinning my arms above my head. He starts kissing down my neck, onto my chest, and then he picks me up and I wrap my legs around his waist. Things get hot and heavy and, before I know it, we are having sex against a wall, my legs wrapped around him.

I have to bite my lip because there are people just outside the door. His big strong arms are holding me up, and sweat is pouring off us like water. What makes it more intense is that we could be caught at any time. Best. Workout. Ever.

Viv

Viv is a heterosexual woman in her thirties. She is married and lives in a rural area. She has a high sex drive and fanta-sizes about sex with other women, threesomes with men and with women, group sex, sex with her boss and watching some-one masturbate. She currently works as a cleaner in someone's house and this fantasy is about her employers.

I'm working away, polishing the bedside lockers, when I feel someone behind me. The next thing I know, I feel a hand at my pussy. I turn around and my employer is there, wearing only her sexy nightgown. I don't know what to do – whether to take off or stay. I'm rooted to the spot, and she whispers in my ear, 'I want to lick your pussy.' I just say, 'Oh!' and get a strange feeling in between my legs. She helps me get naked, and we are on the bed. She is sucking my breasts and I am getting hotter by the second down below. Just as she is going down to my clit, I hear her husband say, 'What's hap-pening here?' She turns around and says, 'Do you want to join in?' My eyes nearly pop out of my head as he quickly gets out of his clothes, saying, 'Get me ready for her.' She starts sucking him off while still playing with my pussy. I am so wet I could cum already.

She stops, and he turns to me and says, 'Do you want some of this?' His penis looks so big I think it will break me. I just nod and wait for the pain. It hurts, but it's pleasurable at the same time. She sucks my nipples and kisses me. I'm so horny – I start saying that I'm going to cum. He pulls out and starts fucking his wife and I am left feeling empty, so I start licking her nipples and kissing them both. She starts playing with my pussy and then we all cum together.

I am completely wrecked. He gets dressed, and we just lie there. She says, 'This employee-boss relationship is going to be good from now on.' I just smile.

Koko

Koko is a bisexual woman in her thirties. She lives in rural Ireland and is single. She has a high sex drive, and regularly reads erotica. She fantasizes all the time and, at the moment, she fantasizes a lot about someone she works with.

I'm on a work night out. It's getting near to the time to leave, and I'm drunk in a flirty, confident way. My male boss asks where I'm staying and if he can walk me back to my hotel. He's been flirting with me all night, but I've been ignoring it, and it's driving us both wild. I invite him in and, once I close the door to my room, he pins me against it. He kisses me hard, slipping his tongue into my mouth, biting my lower lip. My clit is throbbing for him after a long evening of him watching me. He feels my hard nipples and teases them with his fingers. I'm running my hands through his dark hair, longing for him to spread my legs and slip his fingers deep into my warm, slippery pussy. He eventually drops to his knees, pushes my legs apart and teases me with his nose against my panties. He pulls them to one side and slips his tongue against my bulging clit. Sheer pleasure and intense bliss wash over me, and my legs buckle. I reach for his trousers and his cock is hard. I grab it, feeling it bursting to be inside me, to fill me up. I start moaning and breathing heavily. He's enjoying every stroke.

While we explore one another, my female friend gets back from the club and finds us mid-session. She's surprised that we don't stop, and starts giggling to see us enjoying one another. She takes off her top, exposing her pert, hard nipples, and sits on the bed watching as we lick and taste one another. She invites us over to the bed, where she starts biting my nipples. He's still hard and I need him fucking me. My friend lies on her back, and spreads her legs, exposing her sexy waxed pussy, and I'm bent over on my knees with him still licking me. The feeling is amazing. I slip two fingers inside her. She's so wet, I can tell she's incredibly horny. I massage her clit, wanting to taste it and lick her to orgasm. I'm bent over doggy style and He slips his hard cock inside of me. His hardness filling me up is so good. I let out a gasp and scream with satisfaction. I'm licking my friend, and she writhes with pleasure. He's fucking me hard from behind, moaning as he starts to cum. I'm so turned on now that I start to cum while I bring my friend to orgasm as well. A dirty night, but a job well done.

Marcushie

Marcushie is a heterosexual woman in her forties. She has a high sex drive. She considers herself to be a very good lover. Women never feature in her fantasies, but she regularly fantasizes about a particular priest.

I work as a cleaner in a priest's house. One day I'm working away and this tall – not quite good-looking, but definitely sexy – priest dressed in his long, black robes walks towards the cupboard to get something. I'm already in there getting my cleaning products, and he sees me bending down. He gently brushes past my bottom and I feel the sexual tension. I let him know that I like it by smiling sexily at him, so he starts to feel my bottom. I am really turned on, but I pretend not to be, so I bend down again but he knows I want him to feel me again. I'm in charge.

He asks me can he please just feel one of my breasts and I say, 'Okay, but that's it.' He lifts me up onto a table and puts his hand on my breast, getting very excited. Very quickly, my nipples get hard. He wants to touch the other one. I pretend to not want him to. I want him to beg. Then I give in and let him remove my top and bra. He is like a wild animal, rubbing my breasts with his big hands.

'Please let me suck them,' he says.

So I give in, mad for it, wanting more of him. I'm getting so wet that my vagina is thumping. I put my hand on his penis, it's huge and I'm really crazy for it by now. I start to rub his massive penis and it's getting very wet.

'Please lick it,' he begs. I say no, but he keeps asking, and finally, begging, so I give in. I lick it and suck it till he is going crazy. I don't want him to take his off robes, as I'm so turned on by them. He takes the rest of my clothes off, leaving on the robes. At this point I am totally naked on a table in an unlocked cupboard, and anybody could walk in. This is turning me on even more. He is begging me now to let him put his massive penis in my vagina. I keep saying no, talking to him like he is a little boy, until I finally give in. He grabs me by my hips and pulls me towards him.

I tell him to go slowly, because I want to feel every inch of it going in. He obeys me and starts off slowly. I'm moaning, wanting to scream, letting out yelps, and my breathing is very heavy. I tell him I want every inch and to give me all he has. He starts to bang me very, very hard, making the table shake. I tell him to hurry before someone comes in. I'm starting to cum. I feel the heat. I'm going crazy, telling him, 'Don't stop now, don't you dare stop now, give me more, I want it all!' He goes faster. He starts telling me he is going to cum. I tell him, 'Don't you cum now, don't you cum!' and, with that, I have a massive, explosive orgasm, unlike anything I have ever felt before. He comes like a crazy man.

We stop to catch our breath. I put my clothes back on, telling him that this will never happen again, knowing that I can't wait for the next time. He leaves fully dressed in his robes, like nothing ever happened.

Dee

Dee is a heterosexual woman in her late teens or twenties. She has a high sex drive. Women have featured in her fantasies, as have threesomes with men and women. She has also fantasized about group sex, sex with strangers, domination, watching people masturbate and being watched.

My fantasy takes place in a school setting. It's a teacher-student scene. I am the student. I'm wearing a normal uniform, nothing too sexy, just a kilt, shirt and socks. And sexy underwear underneath. I begin by raising my hand and asking for help. The teacher tries to explain, but I still can't understand. I turn towards him and look into his eyes, then down at his bulge. He is doing the same to me, but with my boobs. He says that he could help me after school with one-to-one time. Then I say that we could just do that now, and he leans in and kisses me passionately, fondles my boobs, rubs my clit. You know the rest.

Gang Bangs

Isabelle

Isabelle is a heterosexual woman in her late teens or twenties. She always used to fantasize about her ex, with whom she'd had amazing sex. Sometimes she fantasizes about men she vaguely knows and doesn't necessarily find attractive. From time to time, women have featured in her fantasies.

I am outdoors somewhere, in a park or near the river, and my wrists are tied up to a fence. I have a blindfold on. Whoever has led me there (a boyfriend or whoever I'm currently crushing on) I trust completely. They come up behind me and start caressing my back and my ass, fondling my breasts, lifting up my skirt. Then I begin to feel other hands. There is another person, maybe more than one, I can't tell. This is a surprise. I thought it was going to be just the two of us.

The other hands start to undress me, touching and rubbing and caressing me all the time. I am moaning and moving my hips gently to a rhythm. They don't fully undress me, leaving my bra and knickers maybe. There are mouths sucking my nipples, rubbing my clit and stroking my ass. I hear their voices too, but don't recognise anyone. Then one guy is entering me from behind, I feel other erections pressing up against me, and breasts too. I am given a breast to suck while I am being fucked from behind. Then that man pulls out and another enters. There too many of them to know how many are touching me or fucking me. I am orgasming over and over, moaning and bucking and twisting my body in their hands, all the while tied up and unable to do anything.

Pauline

Pauline is a bisexual woman in her late teens or twenties. She mostly fantasizes when she is alone. The object of her fantasies depends on her mood – it varies from a stranger to her partner to fictional characters in books, films or games.

I have many sexual fantasies. The fantasy that I decide to enjoy does vary from day today. This one begins with me as a prostitute in a red-light district. I work from a window, and this particular night I look damn good, rocking a high ponytail, an insanely short pleated skirt and a very fitted plain white dress shirt, with a few buttons undone to accentuate my ample cleavage.

Without warning, a man in a business suit enters my compartment. Without a word, he grabs me forcefully and backs me against the wall, ripping my shirt fully open. Passers-by start to notice when the buttons of my shirt tap against the glass. The client proceeds to choke me and, running his other hand down my chest, opens my front-clasped bra with one pinch. His hand continues its descent, lower and lower, until the touch of his skin sparks electricity on the side of my abdomen. He undoes his trousers and they drop to the floor. One more fluid movement has his erect penis protruding from over the elastic of his boxers. He has both hands on my ass, pulling me up onto him, forcing himself inside my pussy, my panties brushed to the side to allow him access. My legs envelop his waist. Every part of me aches for his skin. He calls me a dirty whore and slaps my ass, hard, before moving his hand to the back of my neck and gripping it firmly, guiding my actions.

My ecstasy builds as I see that a few of the voyeurs have begun to play with themselves, and even with each other. The glass disappears from the window as I beckon them in. One of the men takes off his pants and, still rubbing his cock, drops to his knees and begins to lick my client's asshole. I continue to slide up and down along his shaft as he groans in pleasure and backs away from the wall and further into the male voyeur's control. A woman begins to fondle my breasts and tempts another to join her. Together, they tweak, nip and lick my nipples with one hand each, and with their other hands begin to play with each other's clits, occasionally brushing against my ass.

The client's grip on my neck gets firmer, and suddenly he decides to rip me off of him and throw me, face-first, onto a table. There is a deafening crack as he slaps my ass cheek once more. I cry out in agony and he bends over me, his erection pulsing as it presses against my back. He grabs my ponytail in one hand and uses the other to pinch my cheeks together and make me look at him.

'You're a filthy fucking slut, nothing but a cheap whore,' he announces.

He throws my face out of his hand, clutches his penis and thrusts it deep inside my asshole. My howl makes him pull harder on my ponytail. The male voyeur smirks and spits on his hand to wet his cock before gently easing it into my client's asshole. The female voyeurs are too busy 69-ing to care what happens in our corner of the room. I can feel my toes begin to tingle.

I blush thinking about this scenario. Without me realising, my hand begins to rub my clit; I can feel the warmth beginning to take over. One of the female voyeurs begins to orgasm, and she squirts so hard that it splashes my ass. My client smirks and, with one final thrust, ejaculates into my anus. It's too much for me to handle; a gasp escapes my lips as I shudder with bliss.

Joanne

Joanne is a heterosexual woman in her late teens or twenties. She has submitted several fantasies for this book. Her fantasies are varied and include sex with other women, voyeurism, threesomes, group sex and sex with strangers. She is single and has a high sex drive.

My fantasy is to go to a really upmarket sex party. I imagine it in an opulent old Georgian house with velvet curtains, plush fabrics and so on. Trust my fantasy to include the soft furnishings. Anyway, I imagine it to be a labyrinth of rooms and, in each room, there are beautiful people indulging in all manner of sexual acts, writhing in pleasure. I imagine walking through the house and lying on the floor, joining in the fun. I like the idea of everyone touching everyone: the sights, the sounds and the actual feelings. I've never actually been with another woman, but I do fantasise about it in this scenario. I love the idea of a number of people pleasuring me at the same time and me reciprocating. I want someone going down on me, another person fondling my breasts and perhaps another person dangling their breasts in my face. That's it really.

Nancy

Nancy is a heterosexual woman in her thirties. She thinks that she is a pretty good lover and has a very high sex drive. Her fantasies often include an ex-lover. He was married and the affair went on for eight years. The sex was spectacular but the relationship ended badly. She continues to think about him a lot. She also fantasizes sometimes about sex with other women.

One of my many sexual fantasies is to be gang-banged. I love to be dominated. The thought of being blindfolded and degraded in front of total strangers arouses me to levels that I have never and may never achieve in my lifetime. In my fantasy, I enter a room with six to eight men and am blindfolded, groped, touched, kissed and licked, with no control over, or knowledge of, who is doing it. My hands are tied above my head. I can hear men around me and feel them playing with me before they each enter me and use me as they please. I am pleasured by only one or two of them but the others simply pleasure themselves without a care for my needs. Men force themselves into my mouth, telling me to take it like a slut, spanking my ass and smacking themselves onto my face. I can hear them moan as they release themselves over my breasts and face. In my mind, this is ultimate filth, and is in stark contrast to my everyday life. This same fantasy can also place me at a swinger'sparty or sex party involving both men and women, being pleasured by men and women, with them dominating me again and again.

Jennifer

Jennifer is a bisexual woman in her thirties. She lives in rural Ireland. She has a very high sex drive. She reads erotica and fantasizes when alone as well as before and during sex.

My partner and I see a couple at the bar. Eye contact between all four of us is continuous. We eventually edge our way closer and start a conversation. There's red-hot attraction in the air. Drinks are flowing, along with my juices. We decide to bring our drinks to our rooms. We all get into the elevator, where the beautiful lady locks lips with me while the guys stand there and enjoy. We can't get into the room quickly enough. Clothes are torn off, soft lips are on mine while two other sets of hungry lips are all over my body. She moves down my body, licking and kissing, until she hits the spot and I'm squirming in pleasure. My man gets in behind her and starts licking to his heart's content. Meanwhile, her man has presented my mouth with his beautiful cock. I eagerly oblige. She's gasping, and I'm moaning as a familiar feeling builds up inside of me.

Georgina

Georgina is a lesbian in her late teens or twenties. She lives in rural Ireland and is currently single. She usually fantasizes when she is alone, about whoever she has a crush on at the time.

My biggest fantasy is group sex, but only women. It has always been a fantasy of mine, from when I was about twelve. A group of women on a bed all arousing each other just sounds awesome, and like something I want to participate in. Group sex nights exist in Ireland, but only mixed gender. Can we kick the men out for one night, Ireland?

Bella

Bella is a heterosexual woman in her late teens or twenties. She is just coming out of a relationship. She has a high sex drive and considers herself to be a good lover. She fantasizes about many different, mostly faceless, strangers. Usually there is more than one person in her fantasy. When she fantasizes about the person she's sleeping with at the time, it's normally just about him.

I have many fantasies consisting of many different and varied scenarios, dynamics and roles. The following fantasy is my favourite, and I've developed it a lot over the years.

I am unhappily married to a rich, bitter, blind man in a huge old Georgian house. It is before women had rights and freedom to choose for themselves, and I feel a sense of being completely isolated, lost and trapped. Life has little meaning, yet I feel a sense of longing and go in search of it within the house.

We have staff and, at dinner, sit at a long dining room table. One evening we are sitting for dinner, myself and my blind, stern husband, the staff standing around to wait on us. There is a cold, tense silence, and I start to look at my staff. I look back into the nothingness and cry. My husband ignores my sobs. One of the male staff comes around to the back of my chair and wraps his hand around the back of my neck so that I turn my face to look up at his. He holds my gaze. My husband, unaware of what is happening, carries on eating.

I feel uneasy: scared but also thrilled. There is a waitress standing behind my husband, watching what is happening.

As the waiter holds my gaze, he slowly moves his head towards me and, with perfect timing, quietly moves his other hand inside of my shirt and down towards my breasts. His lips touch mine ever so gently and our tongues slip into each other's mouths, gently rubbing each other. His hand cups my whole breast, and he slowly moves it over towards the other, gently doing the same thing, rubbing from one to the next, and brushing my nipples. Forgetting where I am, I accidentally let out a slight moan. We pause in fear, his hand on my breast, mouth on my mouth, tongue gently touching my tongue.

'What was that?' My husband asks. I pull away.

'Nothing,' I say.

The female waiter walks towards the back of my husband's chair, looks at me with a deviant smile and puts a finger to her lips . . . *Ssshhh!* I knowingly smile back.

'Be quiet and touch me', I say to my husband The waitress then sits on his lap, pretending to be me, and rubs her ass on his crotch, takes his hands around to her breasts and moans. He automatically engages with her, thinking he will have me.

The waiter and I go back to our previous positions, only more deeply engaged now. He opens my shirt, stands me up, pulls down my skirt and sits me back down. Then he continues to rub my breasts, kissing me all the time. His hands move down to my stomach, and then slowly to my thighs. His gentle fingertips brush over my vagina, but my knickers are still on. He spreads my legs apart, brushes along my inner thigh, kisses my neck. He then comes around in front of me, I open the buckle of his pants and he exposes his large, erect cock, holding it in front of me.

I lick along the shaft, kissing and licking the tip, until it is all wet with my saliva, while he plays with my breasts, constantly maintaining eye contact with me. He then pulls me up, sits on my chair and pulls me back onto him, my ass rubbing against his hard cock. I stare at my husband and the other girl, who are dry humping. Her breasts are big and he is rubbing them all over, moving them up and down. This turns me on. I am dying to feel his huge cock inside my wet, throbbing vagina. The girl slowly takes off her skirt and knickers, and my husband rubs her ass. She sits back down on him and puts his cock inside her. She pulls his hands back onto her breasts, still facing me. Our eyes are locked. She has a smug, warm smile on her face. She has a glint in her eye as if she knows the gift she is giving me, as if she knows and understands my isolation and sadness and, like me, is writhing in pleasure at defying the power!

The man I am on now has his fingers all over me, gently rubbing my vagina inside the lips, back and forth over my clit. I lift myself slightly forward, and he moves my knickers to the side and slowly slips his cock inside me. I move back onto him, rubbing him into me slowly yet hard and deep. He kisses my neck, rubbing my breasts with one hand and my clit with the other, and I grind my body in absolute pleasure into his. As I cum, he cums, and the girl gets off my husband, walks over to us sits on me and kisses me on the lips.

'I hadn't finished! Where have you gone?' My husband says.

I lie there still, basking in pleasure. In that moment, there is connection, intensity and peace, and my whole body feels bliss.

Writing this turned me on more than when I imagine it in my mind. It's been a ery interesting experience for me. I hope it doesn't bore the reader though.

Heidi

Heidi is a heterosexual woman in her thirties. This is the second fantasy she has submitted for this book. She is separated and lives in rural Ireland. She has a very high sex drive and considers herself to be a very good lover.

One of my most frequent, most secret fantasies is one in which I have sex with more than one man – lots of men, in fact. I am on a large bed in a room, probably a hotel, and all around the bed there are naked men – five or six of them. I invite them onto the bed with me, two or three at a time. The other guys wait patiently, stroking their cocks; watching them out of the corner of my eye turns me on. I love knowing that they want me. I have sex with them all, one or two or maybe even three at a time.

I have only confessed this fantasy to one other living soul until now. If I was a man, it would probably be okay – I'd be a stud if I had sex with five or six women in one go, but because I'm a woman, society would no doubt see me as a slut. And while I'd like to think that I am absolutely not and I am totally comfortable with my sexuality, I am obviously ashamed of this thought, otherwise it would not be a secret. Right?

I watched a TV programme recently called 'Sex Party Secrets'. It reminded me of *Eyes Wide Shut*, which I saw years ago. I watched it with my then husband, my sister and my brother-in-law. We were two couples in our twenties and thirties. We were young, fit and healthy and enjoying active sex lives. Well, my husband and I were – I presume that they were too. However, it was uncomfortable watching the big sex party scene with them in their living room. There was some low murmuring from the lads, and each of us was shifting uncomfortably in our seat – not daring to make eye contact with the others. It was like watching it with our parents! We never even spoke about it afterwards.

I remember the masquerade ball: the masks, the well-dressed, sexy party guests, the animalistic debauchery of that scene where Tom Cruise is walking through the mansion and everyone around him is fucking. I found it so hot. I vowed to myself then that I'd do that one day. That TV programme I saw just re-enforced the idea. I've applied for membership at some of these clubs in London.

I think it would be fair to say that group sex is one of my favourite fantasies. Or, at the very least, sex with more than one person at a time. However, I am now in my thirties and I have not yet succeeded in making it happen. I would not have described myself as bisexual. I am curious about having sex with another woman, but I have not done it. So I doubt I am. Or I would have done something about it, no?

Recently, on a drunken night out with my rugby team, I snogged one of my (straight) teammates. Now, I know what you are thinking: 'So what, that happens all the time with female rugby players.' Sorry to burst your bubble, but it doesn't.

Well, we slightly more than snogged. There was some boob action too – nipple-sucking down a quiet road behind the pub. She instigated it. One of our other teammates disturbed us, and proceedings were halted. Who knows what might have happened next? We returned to the pub and carried on like nothing had happened. Needless to say the next morning, neither of us mentioned it.

I find myself fantasizing about her now. About me, her and this guy I know, all of us exploring, teasing and pleasuring one another. I know he would be absolutely up for it, but I have no idea how to even broach the subject with her – keen and all as she was that night. Perhaps I'll wait until the end of the season to ask her.

Three Is Not a Crowd

Sal

Sal is a heterosexual woman in her thirties. She usually fantasizes when she is alone. The object of her fantasy is always a stranger or someone she's just met. They are making overt sexual comments about her body, usually her breasts. She allows the stranger to touch them, and this arouses her. Sometimes it is a man, sometimes a woman and sometimes a couple.

I am away on holidays with my husband. We are in some type of resort and just lounging around by the pool. I keep seeing another couple nearby and am aware of the girl looking at me in my bikini. One day, when my husband has gone off to the shops, she approaches me at a secluded spot by the pool. We start chit-chatting, and she says she thinks my body looks smoking hot. She says that she and her partner were discussing my breasts and she reckoned I'd had a boob job. I tell her that I'm all-natural and she is amazed. In a very matter-of-fact way, she asks for a feel. I'm a bit taken aback but don't want to appear prudish, so I say yes. She slips her hand under my bikini top and starts massaging my breasts. Instantly, my nipples are erect and I'm feeling very turned on. She gets really involved and she knows I'm into it too. Suddenly, I am aware of her boyfriend coming over, and she says he won't mind, as long as he can watch. I agree, as him watching me seems like such a turn-on as well.

My top is gone, and her boyfriend watches raptly as she starts sucking and licking my breasts. I'm breathing hard: am so horny. I can't believe what's happening. She says she wants to make me cum, so I let her slip off my bottoms and she starts to finger me. Her boyfriend goes behind her and pulls down her bikini bottoms and starts to fuck her. All the while he is staring at me, mouthing that he wants to fuck me too. I nod, because I want him to. Then she moves back up to my breasts, and he moves around to me and starts to fuck me hard. After we finish, we go our separate ways, but still watch each other around the pool with lustful looks.

Lara

Lara is a heterosexual woman in her thirties. She rates herself as a good lover and often fantasizes about her tall, gorgeous husband. However, women also feature in her fantasies from time to time, as do force fantasies, threesomes, group sex and domination.

The scenario I always think about when I'm masturbating is me with a man and a woman. I'm wearing a very sexy, tight leather outfit with the chest part missing. The woman in my fantasy is blonde and has big breasts. She is standing in front of me, kissing me. She is naked, and we are touching each other. She sucks on my breasts while I touch hers. The man comes up behind me and enters me with a forceful thrust. I'm so excited and wet. The woman comes closer and I suck wildly on her breasts, making her moan and groan while she masturbates. The man is pounding me from behind so hard that he comes. He lies there and watches the woman and me caressing and kissing each other all over, turning each other on. The man then puts me on my back and goes down on me, making me cum quick and hard, then turns to the woman and does the same with her.

Lynn

Lynn is a heterosexual woman in her thirties. She fantasizes when she is alone, as well as before and during sex. She reads erotica regularly and her fantasies are varied, though they never include women. The man she fantasizes about is usually a great lover but quite submissive in bed.

In my fantasy, my husband is aware that a male friend of ours secretly wants me. He finds the friend making a pass at me in a bar and decides to show him that he never has a chance with me. My husband pulls me into a dark, empty storeroom, and the friend follows. He tells the friend that he will allow him to watch once, and prove that he never stands a chance with me. My husband, who is normally a submissive lover, tells me to get on my knees. I resist at first, but find myself very turned on. I am told to unzip his pants and take him in my mouth. All the while, our friend is watching, speechless.

My husband then lifts up my dress, enters me from behind and tells our friend that he can touch himself, but he must always remember that he will never get his hands on me. The friend is rubbing himself, watching us. My husband gets caught up in the erotic situation and tells the friend to put his cock in my mouth, and I suck him off as my husband has his wicked way with me. Afterwards, my husband tells the that friend if he ever catches him near me again, he will ruin him.

Alex

Alex is a lesbian in her thirties. She considers herself to be a very good lover and has a very high sex drive. She fantasizes a lot, and it's usually about her gorgeous and sexy partner, with whom she has been for over a decade.

I have a number of different fantasies, but there are a couple of recurring ones that never go away. In one of them, I'm coming home after a long day in work, and as I open the door of the house, I can hear moans coming from the bedroom. Thinking that I'm going to catch my partner masturbating, I hurry upstairs, only to see her going down on a mutual friend, who I have a secret 'thing' for. I'm not angry, particularly when they both turn to me and welcome me into the bed. Both have absolutely stunning asses, which is a big turn-on for me. They take charge, making me lick them everywhere, including their assholes. They are wet, wet for me, and it's incredible.

Lola

Lola is a heterosexual woman in her thirties. She has a very high sex drive and mostly fantasizes when she is alone. She sometimes fantasizes about people she knows or ex-lovers. She has submitted more than one fantasy for this book.

This fantasy starts out with me meeting an old fling called Xavier from years ago. In my fantasy, the feelings have never really left either of us, even though it was a long time ago. I plan a visit overseas, and we arrange to meet on the beach where we used to hang out. The heat between us is intoxicating and increasingly intense. Xavier introduces me to his friend James who is absolutely gorgeous. We get chatting. Xavier says he wants to go for a quick surf and will be back soon. After an hour or so of flirting outrageously with one another, I ask James to put sun-cream on my back. I lie down and he starts to massage cream all over me. There are other people on the beach, but they are not too close by.

James lies down beside me and starts rubbing the cream behind my bikini lines, moving his hands lower and lower and lower. After a few minutes, he moves closer to me and slides his fingers inside me, slowly to start with, but then more quickly. I haven't had sex in a long time, and this feeling is long overdue. It feels nearly too good. James and I are spooning and I lean backwards to kiss him. We have the slowest, smoochiest, sexiest French kiss of my life. I feel like I'm floating and have gone to heaven.

I look over and catch a couple of guys looking at us. I don't mind. It makes me even more horny. They start to touch themselves. Xavier then starts calling my name as he comes back up the beach, dripping wet. He takes off his wetsuit half-way, exposing his extremely fit physique. I stand up to greet him and wrap my arms around him. I kiss him so hard that he nearly falls backwards. Xavier asks what we have been doing. I tell him that he had wanted James and I to get to know each other, so we did. I ask him to join us on the mat.

Xavier takes off his wetsuit, I lean over to kiss James again and he starts to take my breast out of my bikini top and roll my nipple with his two forefingers. I cannot believe how wet I am again. Xavier starts to rub my bum with his dick – through my bikini bottoms – and then pulls them down to my knees. I lean back then and we kiss very intimately, slowly and sensually, for what seems like forever. He bends down and puts his head between my legs and starts to lick me slowly. He gets faster and starts to push his fingers inside my pussy. I am so wet. He starts to massage my bum again and, while licking me, puts his little finger up my bum. It feels exquisite. I am almost about to cum, when he changes position so that he is inside me from behind and James starts to suck my nipples. It doesn't take long then, and I explode.

Jessica

Jessica is a heterosexual woman in her thirties. She has a very high sex drive and considers herself to be very good in bed. She regularly reads erotica and mostly fantasizes when she is alone. For over ten years, Jessica has had a fantasy lover with the same features and personality. Last year, she met a man just like him.

My fantasy lover has amazing hazel eyes that you can get lost in. On the days they are a deep dark brown, I know that I am going to hand over control, and allow him bring me to new heights. He is a selfless lover; as long as I have multiple orgasms he is happy. Physically, he is of average height, with a shaved head to hide the bald spots. He is a true gentleman: he holds open the door for me and puts me first all of the time. Even as I type this, I'm getting horny for him. He has a bit of a belly and a double chin. He is open and honest, and likes to talk about everything – just what a girl wants. Best of all, he is now mine. I fantasized about him for about thirteen years, and in November 2014 I found him.

I lost my virginity to a man who liked to experiment in the bedroom. He was a few years older than my eighteen years, but he never pushed or forced me into anything I didn't want to do. We had the most amazing sex life. That relationship came to an end and I subsequently searched for a man who, like my previous lover, was confident and open about his sexuality. I knew that I had a sexy beast within me that was just roaring to get out. I have found this lover I was looking for and, once again, my fantasies have begun to pop up at the most unexpected times.

Throughout my search for 'my perfect man', I had the same fantasy every week for several years. I'm sitting in the jacuzzi, having just finished my morning swim. I am feeling really good about it, having completed two kilometres in thirty-two minutes, a personal best. It releases all the tension from work the previous day. I feel the warm water caressing my skin and soothing my aching muscles. The bubbles skim across my swimsuit, and I can feel my nipples becoming hard from the sensation. I let out a little sigh as I stretch my arms and body. Then I can feel the bubbles hitting my vagina. It's just as well I have a red face from my swim. I smile across at the dark-haired girl who enters the jacuzzi. She is an amazing swimmer, and puts me to shame. We chat a little, and then I head for the changing rooms.

I'm standing under the shower, taking off my swimsuit, allowing my body to feel freedom again. My nipples are still hard and my vagina definitely has extra lubrication. I'm thinking of the dark-haired girl in the jacuzzi. She has an amazing body, toned but with lots of curves. I touch my vagina and can feel my own juices. I take a sneak peak around the showers to check that I am on my own. I flick at my clit and sigh. It's been so long since anyone has touched me there. I turn around facing the wall behind the shower and begin to wash the smell of chlorine off my skin. I'm horny, but I think about my day ahead and start a to-do list.

I can hear someone come into the changing room and I think nothing of it. As I lather my body, I feel a hand touch my back. It washes it for me, moving in a slow circular motion – my shoulders, my lower back, my ass. My crack is covered in suds, but I can feel my vagina getting wetter and wetter. I try to turn around to see who it is, but I am stopped and told to keep looking and leaning against the wall. At this point, the automatic button on the shower has popped so the shower has turned off.

I hear a woman whisper, telling me to open my legs. I comply instantly. She caresses my clit with her fingernail, and licks and kisses my vagina as I lean against the cold tiles. One of her hands pushes my upper back so that my nipples and breasts are flattened against the wall. I'm not sure how much of this I can take.

The next thing I know, she slips one finger into my vagina, saying, 'Oh, you have a very tight pussy.' Then I feel another finger enter me. She moves her fingers in and out, slowly at first, then getting faster and faster. I can feel her naked breasts against my back. She whispers in my ear, 'This is our little secret,' as I cum so hard that my knees buckle and it feels like I have fireworks shooting through my toes.

That is how it used to end. Now that I have found my man it goes further.

Recovering from my orgasm, I turn the shower back on,

and let the hot water soak into my body once again. I can feel someone behind me and I hear my boyfriend's voice, saying that he was starting to get worried about me and he had insisted that they allow him into the ladies' changing area. I turn around in shock. I look at him and can see from the deep brown colour of his eyes that he has caught me.

I begin to plead my innocence, but he stops me. He says that he saw the whole thing, and had been touching himself the whole time. He puts his hand to my vagina and says, 'Are you still horny baby?' He grabs my thighs and picks me up, pushes me against the shower wall as his big, hard and oh-so-thick cock rams into my vagina. It doesn't take us long to cum together, breathless, moaning and weak. As I open my eyes I look to the left and see that the girl from the pool is naked, touching herself. We all look at one another agreeing in silence to keep our little secret as we head out of the shower to get dressed.

Maureen

Maureen is a heterosexual woman in her late teens or twenties. She has a very high sex drive and is currently in a relationship. She often fantasizes about a senior co-worker, and women also sometimes feature in her fantasies.

I'm out in a club with my boyfriend, somewhere that nobody knows us, when we start kissing and becoming aroused. We notice a girl nearby who keeps gazing my way. We somehow end up talking to her, and it is clear she is looking for a good time. My boyfriend keeps whispering to me that I'm turning her on. Finally this girl and I start to kiss and caress each other, with my boyfriend sitting in the middle with a massive erection. The three of us quickly escape back to our hotel room, where this girl and I begin to have very sensual foreplay. My boyfriend sits and watches while he rubs his erection. After a long time watching me experimenting with another woman, he finally joins in and I watch him bend her over and have sex with her. It gives me pleasure to watch him. Then, finally, it's my turn, and we cum together as he penetrates me.

Audrey

Audrey is a heterosexual woman in her fifties. She often fantasizes about a female ex-lover. Her fantasies include voyeurism, threesomes, watching someone masturbate, someone watching her and group sex.

I am watching two people having sex. They don't know I am there. I want to be there, sucking on the woman's breasts. I am getting increasingly hot as I hear noises coming from them – sucking, moaning. I have to touch myself, I am so aroused. I am very wet and, when I touch myself, feel an excruciatingly wonderful sensation. I let a noise escape and suddenly the noises from the couple stop, but I cannot. I make eye contact with the woman and she smiles at me, beckoning me towards them. I cannot move as I am so close to coming, and I am also scared too. She comes over and kisses me then, and it is wonderful. She puts her hand down below with mine, and I explode with a feeling that I cannot describe. I collapse, but the man is there to catch me and take me to the bed. They slowly undress me, as I am lost in the most amazing feeling of wellness.

Suddenly I am being kissed again, this time by the man, and my breasts are being caressed and sucked by the woman – heaven. She offers me her breasts and I melt. He slowly moves down and turns me over, with the woman underneath me. He rubs me underneath, and I suck the woman's breasts. She is touching and kissing me from the front while he enters me from behind. I feel the explosion coming again and moan or scream – I don't know which. She is licking me in front and he is pounding into me from behind, and I leave this earth for an unknown time. When I come round, I am lying on my side with her arms around me. She is sucking gently on my nipple and he is above us with a huge erection and I wonder what is coming next.

Anastasia

Anastasia is a heterosexual woman in her late teens or twenties. She has never had a serious relationship. She has submitted more than one fantasy for this book.

My boyfriend and I are in a bedroom with another woman. She has a great figure, with large breasts and blonde hair. We are all naked. I'm on top of my boyfriend and we're having sex. The woman is sitting across the room, watching us.

She gets up and walks toward us and gets on the bed. She places herself on top of my boyfriend's face and he starts licking her. While his dick thrusts into me, the other woman and I start kissing and playing with each other's nipples. She's making me so wet. We both start to cum; we are breathing heavily on each other and moaning. Our bodies are sweaty, and she starts to rub my clit while I grab her breasts. I moan – it's pleasure I have never experienced. We cum at the same time, then lie there naked on the bed before round two begins.

Kym

Kym is a bisexual woman in her forties. She has submitted two great fantasies for this book. She is married and lives in rural Ireland. This fantasy is a memory from a sexy summer in the west of Ireland.

For the summer between my second and third years in college, I got a job in Connemara. I lived above the local pub, and spent each evening in the bar, playing pool and practicing my hopeless Gaeilge. Usually, I was one of two or three women in the crowded bar, and I loved the attention. One night, I hit it off with a fella about my age, Seán. He had wonderful piercing blue eyes. I got quite hot flirting with him in the bar. I was very disappointed when he told me that he had to leave early to meet with his girlfriend. She was seventeen and not allowed to go to the bar. Later that night, after the bar was closed, there was a knock at my door. Seán was there. It turned out he had had a heavy petting session with his girlfriend, but she was just that bit younger than Seán and I, and still a virgin, and he showed up at my door as horny as a rabbit on steroids. Oh Janey Mack, he did all the things to me that he couldn't do with his underage girlfriend – he was insatiable.

After that night it became a habit. Seán would see his girlfriend early in the evening and then knock at my door after midnight or in the early hours of the morning. It was very much a symbiotic relationship, and I was more than happy with 'no strings' sex.

After a couple of weeks, I met another fella in the pub downstairs. He also had piercing blue eyes, but was much bigger and more muscly than Seán. I wasn't that attracted to him as a person. We had nothing in common, but that body was like something I had never seen. This fella Dathaí would not take no for an answer. He insisted on walking me home, which was out the front door and around the back. *Oh, what the hell*, I thought, and I brought him up.

His bare chest was fantastic – just the right amount of hair, and a super sexy 'treasure trail' disappearing down into his waistband. He had a physical job and was rippling with muscles. Once he got rid of his shirt, I was dripping wet just looking at him and more than eager. What he lacked in technique, he made up for with enthusiasm. I have never met anyone else who could pump a cock into me as furiously as Dathaí (though my hubby comes a close second). In addition to this, he had the stamina to last, and could bring me to several orgasms doing little else. He was so strong that he could just flip me over or pick me up and use me as his sex toy anyway he pleased. I'm five foot nine, so I'm not exactly light and petite. The fact that he was totally in control was a huge turn-on. Just thinking about it now, twenty years later, gets me wet. Of course, I had to get Dathaí out of the flat by 12:30 AM, when Seán was going to come knocking. I made up some excuse for him not to stay the night and let Seán in about thirty minutes later. I fucked Seán as usual that night and said nothing about Dathaí. I was turning into a filthy nymphomaniac!

The next day at work I was still sore from the pounding the two lads had given me the night before. While I was thinking about the evening's escapades I was getting horny all over again. I couldn't believe I was such a slut. *Feck it*, I thought. *Nobody knows me here and I will be gone again in a few weeks. I have nothing to lose.* Dathaí was in the bar again that evening and was looking for a repeat of the previous night. I had already predicted this might happen, and even hoped that it would. I wanted more of both Seán and Dathaí. I had another fantastic night of sex with the lads.

On the third night, Seán turned up at the bar while I was talking to Dathaí. I panicked as Seán came right over to us. 'Hi Dathaí,' he said casually and sat down. *Oh fuck*, I thought, *of course they know each other, it's a small town, how could I be so stupid?* I was worried that I would upset them, or even break a lifelong friendship. Thankfully, Seán came to my rescue. He asked Dathaí to introduce us and pretended not to know me. He had his steady girlfriend and couldn't risk losing her by admitting his relationship with me. So there I sat, chatting with my two lovers, one on either side.

After Sean left to meet with his girlfriend, Dathaí insisted on coming up to my flat. I felt bad and wanted to talk with Seán first, to make sure that he wasn't pissed off at me for being with his friend, but Dathaí was physically forceful – not in a negative, violent way, he was just so hot and horny. I couldn't help but respond. Once Dathaí left, I wondered if Seán was going to come that night, or if I would ever have any more nocturnal visits from him again, now that he knew I was shagging his friend.

But he arrived as usual. Then he asked me how long I had been fucking his brother. Of course, those piercing blue eyes! How could I not have guessed? After some cringing and embarrassment on my side, it turned out that Seán was happy enough for us to continue. He needed some release from the way his girlfriend got him so turned on. We agreed not to tell Dathaí, to save him from any hurt. The last couple of weeks of the summer continued with my two lovers visiting me each night. I would just leave the door unlocked after Dathaí left and Seán would let himself in. He would often wake me up by sucking on my nipples or licking my sore pussy better following Dathaí's vicious fucking.

On my last night before leaving Connemara to return to college, Dathaí and I were hard at it. I was on all fours facing the door while Dathaí was hammering me doggy style. Then the door opened a crack. It was Seán, and he was watching us! Oh God, but I had never felt so hot. How could little old me have such an effect on two men? But, as

I said, I think there was a real lack of young women in the area, and most were not as willing as me. Dathaí must have heard something because he stopped.

'Tar isteach Seán,' he said calmly.

I held my breath, silently waiting for the two to start fighting. But Dathaí stayed in me gripping my hips tightly and Seán entered the room. It looked like I wasn't the only one who couldn't say no to Dathaí. Seán was naked, with a raging erection glistening with pre-cum, and had evidently been masturbating while watching us. Dathaí then just continued with his relentless pounding. I must have looked a sight. My tits were hanging down and bouncing wildly. Seán walked up to me and stuck his cock in my mouth, and I took it willingly. I felt like such a dirty cock-loving whore. It was all so wrong, but that made it a bigger turn-on. Fuck it, if the brothers were okay sharing me, then I was happy to oblige.

Seán fucked my mouth and hung on to my tits as Dathaí fucked my cunt and strummed my clit. It didn't take me long to cum, and Dathaí came soon after. While he lay back and recovered, Seán took his place in my cunt. He flipped me over onto my back and penetrated my slick wet channel almost in one smooth movement. I have wondered ever since if he learned that move from watching his brother and me. It was like he had to reclaim me. His mouth and tongue were everywhere.

The whole scene was made all the hotter by Dathaí watching us. It didn't take long before I was on the verge of cumming again. The next think I knew, Dathaí was at my face and was thrusting his cock into my mouth. We continued like that, with the boys switching places and taking turns until I passed out exhausted and thoroughly fucked.

Though I am very happily married now, I often fantasize about that night of my spit-roasting, sometimes changing the participants to include my hubby.

Abbi

Abbi is a heterosexual woman in her thirties. She describes herself as having a very high sex drive and rates herself as a very good lover. She regularly reads erotica, and usually fantasizes about the last person she slept with or someone she has had good sex with before. Both men and women feature in her fantasies, two of which feature in this book.

Sometimes I am able to have casual sex and sometimes I'm not. By that I mean that I'm sometimes able to do it successfully, and I actually don't want anything else from the person and I don't want it to happen again – or I am unaffected if it turns out that the other person doesn't want it from me again. If it's good enough sex for me to want it again, I am usually somewhat put out when I find that the other person doesn't. I know, who do I think I am? But at other times, my capacity for casual sex becomes something else altogether. Every once in a while, I sleep with someone and it's like reading a great book: I just want someone else to experience it so that I can talk to them about it. I want someone else to fuck him and know how good it is, see if they loved the things that I did, see if they thought it was as spectacular.

I've never gone through with it, but I have fantasized about a casual partner being with a friend of mine. I want it from both sides. I want her to tell me how good he was, that she thought he was great too, how much she loved his cock – assuming that she does. And I want him to tell me what he did to her, every stroke. How he made her cum, what she begged for more of, what he adored about her – assuming that he did. I know the girl I would want and I know the beau.

I'm not sure what about this is so hot for me. I'm not sure why this turns me on, or why I would want this. I know why I would choose the people. The girl is as bold as me and I think she'd enjoy him and I think he'd enjoy being dominated by her instead of dominating me. But who knows. It could all go wrong – they might not be into each other, and that would shatter this fantasy, not to mention an awful situation to have coerced them into. But every time I'm with him, I want it. I want him to talk to me about what he did with her. You never know; it might happen someday.

Aoife

Aoife Brennan is a heterosexual woman in her forties. She loves the idea of threesomes with two hunky men. The man of her fantasies is definitely Michael Fassbender. Aoife is single, and is a writer of erotica alongside lots of other jobs. She has published The Cougar Diaries series. This is an excerpt from one of her books, and a personal fantasy of hers.

Back in Athens the booze had made us sleepy, and we decided to close our eyes for a bit in the quiet of the afternoon. I think I was dozing when I felt a hand creeping between my thighs. I rolled onto my back and opened my eyes. Chris was awake and, as I moved, he sat up and moved down between my legs. He gave Philippe a nudge. 'No sleeping on the job,' he said and Philippe woke up too. He stretched with that sleepy languor of midday naps, and watched Chris licking me. Then he reached out a hand and tweaked my nipple, hard. I sucked in my breath but I felt a direct line between nipple and pussy.

'You have great tits,' he said.

Chris paused for a moment.

'You should taste her pussy,' he said.

'I would, if you weren't so intent on hogging it,' said Philippe, now squeezing my other nipple hard. I reached out and pulled out his thick cock. 'I think Aoife likes cock,' he said.

I smiled my assent. 'I think I do,' I said, pulling firmly as I spoke. Chris looked up again and I chastised him. 'Don't stop now,' I said and he went back to work, his tongue lapping swirls around my clit. He had it down to a fine art; he pushed his fingers into me at the same time, firmly massaging my G spot. Philippe moved and straddled me, feeding his thick cock into my mouth. It was the most amazing feeling. I couldn't see Chris anymore – Philippe's body was acting as a blindfold. Philippe arched his back, pushing his cock deeper into my mouth. He held my throat and pumped rhythmically. My hands were on his chest, sometimes pushing against him if he thrust too deep. All the time, he watched me through hooded, desire-filled eyes.

It was almost too intense. I closed my eyes, for Chris was bringing me to orgasm. I could feel it building and I was not afraid this time. I knew with a certainty, based on nothing more than hope, that my anti-orgasm tumour was well and truly gone. Then Chris changed the motion, and I realised he wanted me to squirt. He was no longer licking me, but firmly stroking his fingers inside me.

'Come to the side and watch this,' he said to Philippe, who obligingly dismounted and knelt by my side. I was glad, for in my growing orgasm, I had found it difficult to give head. I had wanted to bite down hard and did not think Philippe would appreciate that. As it was, finding my mouth free was good, for I could moan with abandon. My right hand held Philippe's cock; it was thick and hard and almost ready to jerk off. My left held my Chris's cock, as he had moved to my other side, but was still fingering me at that steady pace. It was getting to me. I was a two-handed player, and I was about to cum. I was about to squirt. I was the master of my destiny, and I had never felt better. I was positively ambidextrous.

My body twisted and wriggled on the bed as I felt myself about to burst. 'She's coming soon,' said Chris, and the wet noises amplified in the room. I felt my body about to explode. The noises grew: I was the beach, the wave, the ocean. And then I came, loudly. I let go of the two cocks and held my breasts as a waterfall gushed out of me. How could I make such a noise? How could I produce such a waterfall?

I felt like the rainforest. Hell, I was the rainforest, verdant and green and wet.

'Fuck, that is awesome,' said Philippe, who proceeded to cum all over my tits. Chris was not far behind. He pulled at his cock and he too soon jerked across my chest. I was exhausted and horny and spent. 'Fuck, that was awesome,' I repeated, covered in cum, and I ran my fingers down my chest.

Sorcha

Sorcha is a heterosexual woman in her thirties. She describes herself as a fairly good lover with an average sex drive. She occasionally reads erotica and fantasizes either while alone or during sex. She is married, and the object of her desires is usually a stranger but sometimes someone she vaguely knows.

I fantasise about this couple who are acquaintances of mine. I have met them on a number of occasions in social settings, but I don't know either of them very well, and I am surprised when they invite me around for a drink one Friday evening. I arrive at their flat straight from work, wearing an A-line skirt and shirt. He opens the door to me, in what appears to be his gym gear. She is also casual, in jeans and a hoodie. They invite me in. He goes to pour me a drink. We spend about an hour chatting about general nothingness and then the conversation turns to relationships, sex and sexual fantasies. It is obvious that they had been drinking before I arrive and are feeling braver than I. She starts to tell me about her fantasy of being with another woman, and I admit that it is something I have thought about too. He just sits there with a grin on his face. I know where this conversation is going, and yet I am still surprised when they ask. Would I go to bed with them? I ask to take a shower first so that I can get my head around their request.

I step out of their shower and wrap a towel around myself. I walk into the bedroom and they are on the bed. I can see his erection through the thin material of his shorts. They are kissing, and he has opened the zip on her hoodie. She has no bra on, and her tiny breasts are exposed. She is dimpled with gooseflesh, and her nipples are hard. They stop as I enter the room and look at me. I am frightened.

He stands and walks towards me. He kisses me surprisingly gently. He takes my hand and leads me to the bed. He smells of whiskey and the sweet musk of cigarettes. She too smells of whiskey, but under that I can smell the lemon of her shampoo. As I walk, my towel comes loose, and I reach to catch it. A surge of bravery comes over me and I take my hand away and let it drop to the floor. I am very self-conscious. I can feel them looking at me, drinking me in. I sit on the bed, and he starts to kiss my neck and back. Now I am the one with goosebumps.

She leans into me and kisses my mouth. I have never kissed a woman before and it feels strange, different and yet the same. She touches me, runs her hands over me, over my breasts and stomach, and I kiss her back, my bravery and my passion increasing. I push back her hoodie, exposing her more. She reaches to open her jeans and I put my hands between her legs. Her breath catches as I slip my finger into her underwear. I can feel how wet she is. She raises her hips to meet my hand and spreads her legs to let me in. I can feel her husband getting harder behind me. He copies my movements, putting his fingers between my lips, and finding me wet and turned on.

This is amazingly erotic, and while it has literally only been two minutes, I am already close. She is too, and begins to moan. The man takes his cock and starts to tease me with it. He slowly strokes my clit with the tip. When he enters me it is sudden and I gasp, causing his wife to tremble with passion, driving her wild. Her orgasm is slowly building, and I can feel him enjoying her through me. When she does cum, her moans are loud and spasms wrack her body. He hears and sees her enjoyment, and starts to cum too. And so I am left unsatisfied, lying between their spent bodies, their hearts pounding, muscles twitching.

I think they must sense my frustration and she moves to kiss me. She takes my nipple into her mouth and I moan with pleasure. I can see that his dick is still semi-hard. He stands and pulls me towards the edge of the bed then stands over me, gently stroking himself while watching his wife lick my nipples and tease me. He is getting harder by the second. She is on all fours over me, her small breasts dangling in my face. She is more tanned than me, and the contrast of brown on white excites me. Him too, it seems. He enters me from the front and thrusts into me deeply, pelvis on pelvis; it feels amazing. I am slick with perspiration and, as she licks and tastes my salty skin, he brings me to climax.

Nicola

Nicola is a heterosexual woman in her forties. She is married. She has a high sex drive. She likes to think that she is a pretty good lover and often enjoys fantasies about dads she meets through her kids. Other women have also featured in her fantasies.

After I drop my kids to school and return home, I shower and dress in a fluffy bathrobe. The doorbell rings, and two young school dads are standing on my porch wearing tight blue jeans with visible bulges in their crotch areas. Not a word is spoken as they follow me upstairs to my bedroom. I insist on washing them each in the shower, before I suck their huge cocks as they stand against the wall. I bend over and each takes a turn entering me from behind until we all finally explode in a sweaty mess on the rug. They leave, not a word said.

Miriam

Miriam is a heterosexual woman in her late teens or twenties. She regularly fantasizes about an ex-boyfriend. The sex was so good, so passionate, that her mind can't help but wander back to that time together.

It begins in a bedroom around sunrise. The light in the room is soft. I am curled up in the bed, with someone behind me. I can feel his cock hard against my ass and I become instantly wet. His hands caress my breasts as I push back against him, making their way down my body before reaching between my legs, massaging my clit. He pulls my underwear to one side and slides deep inside me. Suddenly the door opens and it is my partner, catching me in bed with this 'stranger' (usually a friend of his).

I look at him, guilty that I'm enjoying another man's cock. I can see he's jealous and angry, but also that his cock is growing harder in his underwear. He makes his way over to the bed and lies down next to us, stroking himself, looking me in the eye as I'm being fucked by someone else. He sucks on my nipples and kisses me. Before long, I'm on all fours. The stranger takes me from behind as my partner's head is between our legs, licking my clit, sometimes accidentally catching a taste of his friend's cock as it pounds in and out of me.

The sensation of his tongue on my clit and a cock inside me brings me over the edge and I cum hard, moaning loudly. The stranger fucks me harder – he is on the edge of coming. I beg him to cum deep inside me, and he does as he's told, filling me. He pulls out and my partner is waiting to clean him up, taking his cock in his mouth, tasting my pussy on it as well as the stranger's cum.

I lie on my back, watching my partner take another guy's cock in his mouth, finding it incredibly arousing. My partner then turns his attention to my pussy, making sure to clean me up too, swallowing the stranger's cum, which drips out of me, and bringing himself to orgasm as he does it.